THE HOSPITALIZED CHILD

Psychosocial Issues

IFI DATA BASE LIBRARY

Recent volumes in the series:

BEHAVIORAL DEVELOPMENT OF NONHUMAN PRIMATES
An Abstracted Bibliography
Faren R. Akins, Gillian S. Mace, John W. Hubbard, and Dianna L. Akins

MASTER TABLES FOR ELECTROMAGNETIC DEPTH SOUNDING INTERPRETATION
Rajni K. Verma

SPECTROSCOPIC REFERENCES TO POLYATOMIC MOLECULES
V. N. Verma

RAPIDLY QUENCHED METALS
A Bibliography, 1973–1979
C. Suryanarayana

MOSFET TECHNOLOGIES
A Comprehensive Bibliography
A. H. Agajanian

PARENT–CHILD SEPARATION
Psychosocial Effects on Development
An Abstracted Bibliography
Faren R. Akins, Dianna L. Akins, and Gillian S. Mace

THE BEREAVED CHILD
Analysis, Education, and Treatment
An Abstracted Bibliography
Gillian S. Mace, Faren R. Akins, and Dianna L. Akins

THE HOSPITALIZED CHILD
Psychosocial Issues
An Abstracted Bibliography
Dianna L. Akins, Gillian S. Mace, and Faren R. Akins

THE HOSPITALIZED CHILD

Psychosocial Issues

An Abstracted Bibliography

Dianna Lyell Akins

University of Arizona
Tucson, Arizona

Gillian S. Mace

San Jose State University
San Jose, California

and

Faren R. Akins

University of Santa Clara
Santa Clara, California

IFI/PLENUM • NEW YORK-WASHINGTON-LONDON

Library of Congress Cataloging in Publication Data

Akins, Dianna L.
The hospitalized child, psychosocial issues.

(IFI data base library)
Bibliography: p.
Includes indexes.
1. Children—Hospital care—Psychological aspects—Abstracts. 2. Children—Hospital care—Social aspects—Abstracts. 3. Sick children—Psychology—Abstracts. 4. Children—Hospital care—Psychological aspects—Bibliography. I. Mace, Gillian S. II. Akins, Faren R. III. Title. IV. Series. [DNLM: 1. Child, Hospitalized—Psychology—Abstracts. ZWS 105.5.H7 A315h]
RJ242.A38 362.1'9892 81-12007
AACR2

ISBN 978-1-4684-9098-5 ISBN 978-1-4684-9096-1 (eBook)
DOI 10.1007/978-1-4684-9096-1

Softcover reprint of the hardcover 1st edition 1981
A Division of Plenum Publishing Corporation
233 Spring Street New York, N.Y. 10013

PREFACE

The Hospitalized Child: Psychosocial Issues is a comprehensive, abstracted bibliography focusing on the behavioral and developmental consequences of short-term, long-term or recurrent hospitalization during childhood and adolescence. The emphasis of this volume is on the psychosocial issues related to the hospital experience/environment, rather than on adaptation to or coping with particular disease states or terminal illness. Publications are included which identify potential problems of hospitalization, coping mechanisms of patients, parents, and staff, and possible solutions. For example, the articles covered in this volume discuss the trauma which may result from the child's separation from mother/family/peers, anxiety over medical procedures, unfamiliarity of the hospital environment, absence from school, restrictions on physical activity, forced dependency and concerns over body image. The search for solutions to adaptation difficulties often results in the creation of new hospital programs. These too are reviewed in this bibliography. Examples include child-life programs, the care-by-parent units, foster grandparent/surrogate mother programs, and hospital or surgical orientation programs. New therapeutic approaches have been attempted in a hospital setting, including bibliotherapy, puppet therapy, play therapy and mutual-story-telling techniques. Each of these innovations is represented in the bibliography. Further, hospital redesign schemes are reviewed, including the feasibility of separate adolescent wards. And finally, modification of hospital policy has been examined, including establishment of liberal visiting privileges, parent rooming-in, day surgery, and improved communication between patient, parent, and hospital staff.

The Hospitalized Child: Psychosocial Issues contains over 500 citations in author-alphabetized and abstracted form. Only English-written books and periodicals are represented. Because of the relative recency of interest in this topic and the current bulk of information, only post-1970 articles are abstracted. A historical section lists over 250 additional materials published between the years 1960-1969. Literature across multiple disciplines was scanned and included. Medicine, nursing, psychology, and social work journals are heavily represented. Abstracts for the publications were obtained from Psychological Abstracts, the original article or were written by the authors of this bibliography. An author and subject index appears at the end of the book. Each citation is assigned one or more subject terms. An additional feature is a "Stop Press" section listing 41 post-1970 articles located after the main text was assembled.

It is the hope of the authors of this volume that this bibliography will prove useful to physicians, nurses, medical social workers, hospital staff, psychologists, researchers and all professionals involved in the area of childhood and adolescent hospitalization.

CONTENTS

BIBLIOGRAPHY

1. Abbas, A., & Rolinson, J. A library of toys. Nursing Times, 1974, 70(15), 564-565.

This article describes the responsibilities and services provided by an Organizer of Play and Training Equipment employed at two large hospitals. The author reports that such a position offers the following positive benefits: (1) Considerable economy has been effected as a result of buying toys in bulk from commercial firms and by enlisting help from public institutions and voluntary organizations. (2) Further economy has been achieved by regular stocktaking and by ensuring that items are only condemned if they cannot be repaired. (3) Patients have an opportunity to play with more appropriate toys and a much wider variety is available to them. (4) The provision of an annual budget ensures that at least a minimum amount is spent each year on this important material. (5) The existence of the organizer and the working parties maintains in the nursing and other departmental staffs an interest in the educational and recreational functions of toys and play equipment. (6) Some volunteers prefer the opportunity of producing equipment which they know will contribute to the benefit of patients.

2. Abbott, N. C., Hansen, P., & Lewis, K. Dress rehearsal for the hospital. American Journal of Nursing, 1970, 70, 2360-2362.

This article describes a program for pediatric patients which attempts to orient them to the hospital. The fears of most of the chidlren encountered were analyzed, and a program to orient well children to a potential hospital experience was instituted. The program was taken to the schools in the Phoenix, Arizona, area, and presented to kindergarten children because they were considered the most vulnerable. The program and the children's responses to what was presented are described. Regardless of which hospital the child is admitted to, the adjustment of children who have participated in the program seems good. The children seem to have fewer anxieties, seem more familiar with their environment, and are generally cooperative. A program to orient the school nurses to the hospital so they can lead this kind of program is being undertaken.

3. Ack, M. Considerations governing the organization of a children's hospital. Journal of the Association for the Care of Children in Hospitals, 1975, 4(1), 27-32.

This article first discusses why it has often been difficult to integrate psychological insights into the practice of medicine and presents some anecdotal statements on the history of mental health efforts to influence institutions. The author then presents a systems analysis of how current hospital programs could be modified to better serve the pediatric patient. Factors such as increased parental participation, increased psychological understanding by staff, and more multidisciplinary approaches to child care are stressed.

4. Ack, M. New perspectives in comprehensive health care for children. Journal of Pediatric Psychology, 1976, 1(4), 9-11.

The total health of the child, including emotional well-being, is emphasized by the Children's Health Center of Minneapolis. To produce such an institution, two areas were dealt with: the psychological sophistication of the staff and the construction or alteration of system factors to allow this psychological sophistication to be manifested. A number of humanizing innovations which have been introduced in this hospital are described, ranging from architecture to the details of the ways in which medical technicians relate to children.

5. Acord, L. T. One five year old boy's use of play. Maternal-Child Nursing Journal, 1980, 9(1), 29-35.

This paper illustrates how one five year old used play to reveal his concerns of intrusive procedures. The study was conducted in a large metropolitan children's hospital. A total of six play interviews was conducted, using a kit of toys representative of items used in hospital and home settings. Four play sessions were held in the hospital, and two sessions were held in the living room of the subject's home. Although the play sessions revealed more than a fear of intrusive procedures, this article is limited to the discussion of this area since it was his major area of concern. There were indications of progression in the direction of mastery of these concerns across the observational sessions as discussed by the author.

6. Adams, M. A. A hospital play program: Helping children with serious illness. American Journal of Orthopsychiatry, 1976, 46(3), 416-424.

Children hospitalized with a life-threatening disease may experience a severely stressful situation that is often confusing, frightening, and anxiety-provoking. The present paper describes a play-therapy program designed to facilitate the expression of these feelings, enhance the child's sense of mastery, foster adaptive behavior, and increase his or her cooperation with medical treatment.

7. Aiken, M. A. Flight. Fight. Or . . . Journal of the Association for the Care of Children in Hospitals, 1978, 7(1), 23-27.

This article describes the efforts of the mother of a hospitalized child to seek treatment reforms from hospital administration. The author outlines some of the changes she and other volunteer parents were able to achieve: (1) children room only with other children, rather than adults; (2) toys were provided for the children to play with; (3) environmental changes were made to make the rooms more colorful and comfortable; (4) hospital tours for children were begun; (5)

volunteer parents stayed as companions for children to decrease isolation; (6) parents may stay overnight; and (7) food may be ordered by parents attending children.

8. Aisenberg, R. B., Wolff, P. H., Rosenthal, A., & Nadas, A. S. Psychological impact of cardiac catheterization. Pediatrics, 1973, 51 (6), 1051-1059.

Fifty children between 4 and 15 years of age were subdivided into three age groups and studied before, during, and after cardiac catheterization. Nearly all of the youngest, but less than half of the oldest patients manifested negative behavioral and intrapsychic changes after catheterization. The behavior patterns of the youngest children were affected specifically in the domains of regression, aggression, affectivity, and attitude. The increase of general and somatic anxiety was equally distributed among older and younger children. Among boys the increase of aggression was typically expressed in physical modes, whereas girls more often responded by verbal aggression. Since children do not perceive cardiac catheterization as an innocuous procedure, and the catheterization experience may, in selected cases, interact with previously existing conditions to produce long-term adverse effect, intervention to protect very young cardiac patients may be advisable. Prophylactic play therapy could be utilized; or where medically feasible, cardiac catheterization could be postponed until later childhood.

9. Al Ageel, M. C. S. Reactions of a hospitalized school-age child to separation and restricted mobility. Maternal-Child Nursing Journal, 1978, 7(3), 163-173.

The purpose of this paper is to describe the reactions of a schoolage girl (Betsy) to an injury and hospitalization which posed a crisis to her and her family. Assessment information and related literature provided insight into Betsy's behaviors and a basis for planning care to assist her in regaining mastery. Over time Betsy was able to realize substantial progress in efforts to regain autonomy in self-care; to achieve cognitive understanding of her situation; to pursue learning; to develop relationships with others, and to be able to play. Through follow-up contacts with Betsy and her family, the nurse-writer was able to witness their successful resolution of the health crisis they faced. Hopefully, that success will increase their ability to use their inner resources in dealing with future problems.

10. Albertini, R. Use of paradoxical injunction with a hospitalized adolescent. Hospital and Community Psychiatry, 1979, 30(3), 163-164.

For the adolescent who undergoes prolonged hospitalization, an imbalance may sometimes occur in the normal independence-dependence struggle. The adolescent may become overly dependent on his new hospital "parents"--the staff. Thus impaired by physical illness, the hospitalized adolescent may assert his independence in ways that are perceived by the hospital staff as defiant and negativistic, thus increasing the likelihood of a struggle for control between patient and staff. This article describes a case study which illustrates the use of paradoxical injunction in dealing with a hospitalized adolescent involved in a power stuggle with the staff. The case shows that paradoxical injunction may prove effective in treating the acting-out hospitalized adolescent by allowing him some measure of control over himself without the hospital staff's having to relinquish all "parental" responsibility. Other approaches may only increase inevitable "parent-child" power struggles.

11. Alcock, D. Hey, what about the kids? The Canadian Nurse, 1977, 73, 38-41.

This article reports a survey of pediatric units throughout Ontario, Canada, undertaken in 1976 to learn more about how these hospitals are equipped to meet the non-clinical needs of the children who are admitted to them. A total of 74 questionnaires were sent to hospitals with more than 20 pediatric beds. A survey base of 50 hospitals was obtained. Findings of this survey were similar to the results of another survey in the Maritime Provinces, and indicate important ways in which hospitals in Canada are failing to provide the facilities, personnel and environment that pediatric patients need. For the most part, pediatric staff seem aware of children's needs but uncertain about the best way of dealing with these concerns. Suggestions are made for the improvement of pediatric care, and the implications of the results discussed.

12. Allen, J. M. Influencing school-age children's concept of hospitalization. *Pediatric Nursing*, 1978, *4*(6), 26-29.

Positive results were obtained from a single program aimed at identifying and modifying children's feelings about the hospital using the mediums of art and play. Preliminary drawings by 30 school-age children, gave evidence of "faulty knowledge," feelings of fear and confusion, and a lack of certainty about the hospital experience. Given an opportunity to confront their concerns by actively playing with the feared items identified in the pictures, several changes were noted in the post-play drawings. The children conveyed a greater sense of confidence, a focus on reality, and a decrease in fear of the unknown. This study seems to support the theory proposed by Plank, Almy, Clatworthy, and others, that play can be used to identify the views of healthy children toward the hospital setting. Art appears to be an effective medium for the expression of such views.

13. Altshuler, A. *Books that help children deal with a hospital experience*. Washington, D. C.: United States Department of Health, Education and Welfare, Publication number (HSA) 78-5224, 1978.

The traumatizing effects of hospitalization in childhood have been widely recognized. Many ideas have been proposed to prepare the child for this experience and to help ease its trauma. One of the potential solutions is the use of children's books. The author has compiled a bibliography of children's books dealing with illness and hospitals. Each book listing is annotated and includes an evaluation based on the quality of the book and the accuracy of the medical information. An asterisk marks books the author believes should be available in a basic library of a children's hospital unit. The information is provided to enable adults to select an appropriate book based on the child's specific illness and age group.

14. Altshuler, A. The adolescent in the general hospital. In J. Howe (Ed.), Nursing care of adolescents. New York: McGraw-Hill Book Company, 1980, 350-368.

Nurses in the hospital setting encounter some adolescents who have a wealth of experience with the health care system as a result of congenital defects or acquired chronic illnesses necessitating frequent and often lengthy hospital stays. Other adolescents are admitted for acute illness, injury, or elective surgery with little knowledge of or prior experience with either the hospital system or the role of being ill. Nursing intervention for both groups needs to be based on a thorough knowledge of and sensitivity to the normal developmental tasks being faced by adolescents, with support for maintaining healthy growth despite the disruptive impact of illness. This chapter presents nursing interventions that facilitate adolescents' adaptation to hospitalization in a growth-producing fashion, regardless of whether they are admitted for an acute health problem or for a chronic condition.

15. Altshuler, A., & Seidl, A. H. Teen meetings: A way to help adolescents cope with hospitalization. MCN: American Journal of Maternal Child Nursing, 1977, 2(6), 348-353.

This article describes how teen meetings can be used to help the adolescent deal with the separation from friends and family. The goals of such meetings are to: (1) convey caring and concern for patients and their needs, feelings, and opinions; (2) provide a setting for teenagers to vent their feelings and share their concerns and fears; (3) foster mutual support for the simultaneous tasks of dealing with hospitalization and illness as well as normal growth and development; (4) provide a forum for conveying acceptance to those who have experienced a major change in body image through burns, amputations, loss of hair, placement in a body cast, or other procedures and conditions; (5) help the adolescents to move more comfortably back into home and school situations; and (6) help teens learn to develop social skills among the group's members. The structure of these groups, the staff's responsibilities, and the effectiveness of the technique are discussed by the authors.

16. Amdall, M. J., Boverman, H., Cohen, S., & Freeman, M. The evolution of a child life therapy program and the impact on a pediatric inpatient service. Journal of the Association for the Care of Children in Hospitals, 1976, 5(2), 4-13.

This paper describes the child life program of the Doernbecher Memorial Hospital, a part of the University of Oregon Health Sciences Center in Portland, Oregon. The authors describe how this program of one to one child care developed and present case studies to illustrate the usefulness of such programs. This report also outlines the results of an extensive evaluation program which demonstrated the strengths of the child life therapy program and pointed out areas of needed expansion.

17. Anderson, M. G. Is this the Liberry? Journal of the Association for the Care of Children in Hospitals, 1981, 9(3), 77-79.

This article discusses how to establish and develop a library in a pediatric hospital. Some suggestions for funding such a project are outlined. The article also discusses the use of a story hour as part of a library program. Some resource material is provided and a discussion of how pediatric hospital libraries can serve the therapeutic needs of children and their families.

18. Andrew, J. M. Recovery from surgery, with and without preparatory instruction, for three coping styles. Journal of Personality and Social Psychology, 1970, 15(3), 223-226.

A stress-reduction method (information giving) was chosen as a possible method to improve recovery from surgery for one personality type--sensitizers--who typically do seek, learn, and use information in their intellectualizing defenses. An opposite-extreme group--avoiders--who seldom use intellectualizing defenses, was expected to improve little; while an intermediate group--neutrals--was expected to improve an intermediate amount. However, results showed learning was unimportant; and that the middle group improved most, recovering in less time and with fewer medications when instructed than when not instructed, while avoiders required more medications when instructed, though not longer time. Sensitizers, expected to show the greatest improvement, did not change. The unexpected results were interpreted in terms of adaptation.

19. Anonymous. Children in hospital. British Medical Journal, 1970, 1(5705), 309-310.

This article briefly reviews some of the historical aspects of problems associated with children in hospitals. Discussion is given to some of the current problems and suggestions made for improving the quality of child care.

20. Anonymous. Children in isolation units. Lancet, 1970, 2(7671), 509.

This article discusses the problems of children hospitalized in isolation units and describes one form of psychological treatment. An experiment in applying the methods of play therapy to children in isolation was started three years ago at St. George's Hospital, in Tooting, London, when, with the help of the Save the Children Fund, a playleader joined the staff of the infectious-disease unit. The result was a notable increase in happiness and activity in the wards; fears that the nursing staff would be left with all the painful tasks while the playleader took over all the pleasant relationships with the children proved groundless. On the contrary, the special skills and methods of the playleader have been disseminated through the wards, and have had a generally beneficial effect on the standard of child care.

21. Anonymous. "Home visits" prepare children for surgery. Journal of the American Medical Association, 1972, 219(6), 680-681.

The hospital comes to the child before the child has to go to the hospital. That is the essence of a combination patient care and training program involving Milwaukee's 580-bed St. Joseph's Hospital and the Marquette University College of Nursing. The training part applies to student nurses; the patients are youngsters of pre-school age. This program was set up in an attempt to answer the question: What can you do for children under five years of age who have to be hospitalized for elective surgery?

22. Anonymous. Fearless of the familiar. Hospitals, 1974, 48(7), 23-26.

This article describes some of the techniques used by staff at the children's Medical and Surgical Center at Johns Hopkins Hospital to help reduce trauma in hospitalized children. When a child is scheduled for admission to the center, the admitting office automatically sends him the Hospital Book, which helps the child learn about the whole process of hospitalization. Simultaneously, the child's parents receive a booklet that describes the special services they may expect and advises them how to support the child before, during, and after hospitalization. After a child is hospitalized, the process of familiarization is continued through the use of the "hospital house," a dollhouse model that lets children see various kinds of hospital equipment in advance. And finally, an attempt is made to surround a child with persons and activities from his environment as much as possible to facilitate emotional stability.

23. Anonymous. Children in hospital--and after. Lancet, 1975, 2 (7936), 649.

This article reports on the health care policy of the Australian Association for the Welfare of Children in Hospital. Briefly, it recommends that: (1) no child shall be taken into hospital unnecessarily, nor kept there any longer than is absolutely essential; (2) parental access to children should not be limited, and facilities for "rooming-in" should be provided; and (3) all the staff should be psychologically trained in the management of children. These recommendations are unexceptionable and most are already in operation in a number of hospitals.

24. Anonymous. A recommended care policy relating to children and their families. Medical Journal of Australia, 1975, 2(supplement 2), 1-16.

This report prepared by the Association for the Welfare of Children in Hospital formulates a number of policy statements regarding the treatment of hospitalized children and their families. Major principles specify that: (1) a child should only be hospitalized if there are clear and unavoidable indications for this; (2) the duration of a hospital stay, particularly for a young child, should be as brief as possible; (3) when health care for the child is necessary within an institution, a close and continuous relationship between the child and the family should be encouraged and maintained wherever possible; (4) every effort should be made to minimize the physical and emotional distress to children and their families; (5) those involved in child care should be chosen with consideration for their special personal attributes such as perception, sensitivity and compassion for young children which will render them more suited to this role; (6) professionals involved in child care should have special training in the unique psychological needs of young children in sickness and in health; (7) the provision of pediatric care, recognizing the physical, emotional and intellectual needs of the child during sickness, provides a special opportunity to help create an informed public opinion about the care of children generally and the relevance of the family; (8) on-going evaluation of policies and programs of care is essential.

25. Anonymous. The young child in hospital: A health hazard? Medical Journal of Australia, 1975, 2(6), 201-202.

The recent upsurge of organizations which cite the welfare of children as their main preoccupation bears testimony to the widespread disquiet about many aspects of child management, particularly in the realm of hospital or other residential care. In Australia, however, although there are clear guidelines laid down for the child's physical needs, it is of significance to note that for the child's emotional needs there are no such guidelines. Such is the concern at this deficiency that the Australian Association for the Welfare of Children in Hospital (AWCH) has produced a document, "A Health Care Policy for Children and Their Families." This "policy document" clarifies what it means to be a young child in hospital and has special relevance for the staff of hospitals. It makes clear recommendations for future action, and it is hoped that Australia will set a standard for the world to follow.

26. Anonymous. Let the children play. Lancet, 1976, 1(7973), 1336.

This article argues that children in hospital should not be deprived of the opportunity to play and should be helped to do so. An important and almost indispensable component of play in hospital is its direction and execution by a particular member of the ward team--the play-worker. Formalization of the professional role of the play-worker and a big increase in their numbers is in order to provide adequately for children in all hospitals. This article reviews the problems which some institutions have had and offers some solutions.

27. Anonymous. A child life program in action. Canadian Nurse, 1977, 73(11), 42-43.

When children or adolescents are ill and hospitalized there is interference with the normal life activities which foster growth and development. There is also stress and anxiety concerned with illness and visits to the hospital. The aim of Child Life programs is to minimize the traumatization of illness and hospitalization and to encourage the continued growth of the child or adolescent--physically, emotionally, intellectually and socially. The Child Life staff also aim to foster involvement in children's activities on the part of all who are in contact with the child and his family. Some of the services and resources made available to patients through the Child Life Program at the Children's Hospital of Eastern Ontario are described in this article.

28. Anonymous. Child life therapists help humanize hospitalization. Hospitals, 1977, 51(21), 14, 16, 20.

The rationale for and the value of child life programs are being recognized by more and more hospitals. The programs in force today differ markedly in specific functions--providing school learning situations, recreation, play experiences, child advocacy, or any combination thereof--but share a common denominator in that they strive to make hospitalization less traumatic for children. One such program, staffed by four salaried child life therapists, has been in effect since 1974 at Doernbecher Memorial Hospital for Children at the University of Oregon Health Sciences Center in Portland, Oregon. An important aspect of the child life therapy program is the training, in-service education, and supervision provided by the department of child psychiatry, which jointly sponsors the program with the department of pediatrics. Another aspect of the ongoing education of the child life therapist is the review and discussion of current literature on children and their care.

29. Anstice, E. Nurse, where's my mommy? Nursing Times, 1970, 66 (48), 1511-1518.

This article reviews some of the problems of children in hospitals including parent-child separation, fear, pain, and neglect. The author also discusses how other family members may be affected by the hospitalization of a child. Discussion is also given to how hospital staffs are affected by such hospitalizations. Some suggestions for dealing with these issues are presented and a plea for mutual support emphasized.

30. Anstice, E. Who'll be mother? Nursing Times, 1973, 69(22), 716-717.

Guided by a convincing body of research, we understand that if the mother cannot be present there must be a mother-substitute figure, one person for the child to become attached to and trust, who can give him the individual love and attention he needs, and act as a buffer between him and the uncertain, sometimes threatening, world around him. The absence of such a person, particularly for any length of time, can cause severe long-term emotional disturbance in the child. This article discusses various mother-substitutes and how they can function to help the hospitalized child. Both the ward sister and the nurse are discussed as possible mother figures.

31. Apt, L., Beckwitt, M. C., & Isenberg, S. Preparing the child and parent for strabismus surgery. American Journal of Ophthalmology, 1973, 75(5), 898-900.

The authors outline a plan to prepare the parent and the strabismic child for hospitalization. The method varies in a manner appropriate with the child's age. After six months of age, separation anxiety is avoided by having the parent "room in" with the child. In addition, the one- to three-year-old child is prepared for hospitalization by approaching the subject through his parents. Little is said about the hospitalization in the presence of the child until several weeks before admission. To prepare the child in this interval, the parents periodically mention the pending hospitalization in a rather casual manner designed to make the child anticipate a pleasurable experience. The authors report that it is advantageous to anticipate and discuss frequently asked questions by the parents to avoid further apprehension. The child's mental stress and anxieties can be reduced to a minimum by this appropriate age-related approach to both the child and parent.

32. Apt, L., Beckwitt, M. C., & Isenberg, S. Emotional aspects of hospitalization of children for strabismus surgery. Annals of Ophthalmology, 1974, 6(1), 11-20.

While any hospitalization and operation is traumatic to child and parent, strabismus surgery, in particular, increases the stress. It is of prime importance to recognize that the level of anxiety in the child is proportional to the level of anxiety in the parents. The physician, therefore, should make a conscious effort to reduce the anxiety of the parents during the treatment of the child. To minimize the separation anxiety prevalent in preschool children, the mother should be encouraged to "live in" with the child during hospitalization and the stay should be kept as brief as possible. In the older patient, anxiety is reduced by an open discussion with parents and child of the impending hospitalization and surgery. In addition, intelligent use of sedation and analgesia, avoidance of simultaneously bandaging both eyes, minimization of injections, and the use of absorbable sutures have all been proven in recent years to reduce stress and anxiety in both parent and child.

33. Asen-Rudbarg Vardaro, J. Preadmission anxiety and mother-child relationships. _Journal of the Association for the Care of Children in Hospitals_, 1978, _7_(2), 8-15.

This investigator analyzed the relationship between 18 mothers' level of anxiety prior to the hospitalization of their children and the preadmission anxiety levels of their children. Anxiety was measured by use of a urine test for an adrenal cortex product (17-Hydroxycorticosteroid), the State-Trait Anxiety Inventory, and the Prehospitalization Behavior Questionnaire. The 18 children, ages 36-66 months, had no previous hospitalizations and were admitted for hernia repair surgery. There were significant postitive correlations between mothers' urinary adrenal-cortex product levels and those of their children and between mothers' state anxiety scores and their children's urinary adrenal-cortex product levels. Mothers' ratings of children's prehospitalization behaviors on the questionnaire did not correlate significantly with mothers' state anxiety scores, with mothers' levels of urinary adrenal-cortex product, or with their children's levels of the adrenal-cortex product. It is concluded that mothers' anxiety levels are related to their children's anxiety levels, and implications for the management of children's anxiety surrounding hospitalization are discussed.

34. Astin, E. W. Self reported fears of hospitalized and non-hospitalized children aged ten to twelve. Maternal-Child Nursing Journal, 1977, 6(1), 17-24.

This study was designed and conducted to identify and explore the relationship between the fears of a sample of non-hospitalized children and a sample of hospitalized children within the same age range of ten to twelve years. One sample of the population included twenty-five children who were admitted to a general hospital. The second sample consisted of twenty-six fifth and sixth graders who attended an elementary school. The instrument was a questionnaire consisting of a checklist of seventy-one items comprising eleven fear categories as developed and revised by Croake. Results showed that there were no significant differences in the number of fears reported overall by the two sample groups, or according to sex and race. The hospitalized children's most frequently mentioned fear types were ranked as political, natural phenomena, ecological and home. For the non-hospitalized children, fear types were ranked as natural phenomena, ecological, political and safety. Fear intensity was measured by a scale of 0 to 4. Hospitalized children had significantly more intense fears than the non-hospitalized children. The implications of these results for the treatment of hospitalized children is discussed.

35. Audette, M. S. The significance of regressive behavior for the hospitalized child. Maternal-Child Nursing Journal, 1974, 3(1), 31-40.

Several implications for the practice of pediatric nursing emerge from the literature on regression and from clinical observations of hospitalized children who use regressive behaviors to cope. One of these implications concerns the adult response to regressive behaviors in hospitalized children. Observations reveal that adults in the hospital, including nurses, were accepting of regressive behavior only when it is exhibited by young toddlers. This is in contradiction to the literature findings which indicate that regression is common and healthy and that it should be expected and accepted in all age groups, including adolescence. Another implication has to do with the advisability of encouraging the parents' presence in order to facilitate the regaining of trust which is necessary for the child to abandon regressive coping. The potential for parents to give such support to their child often seems to be overlooked. A third implication pertains to the potential which nurses have for helping the child avoid the need to regress. They can do this by eliminating or reducing some of the situational stresses. Approaches are suggested to help the child abandon regressive coping.

36. Auer, E. T., Senturia, A. G., Shopper, M., & Biddy, R. L. Congenital heart disease and childhood adjustment. Psychiatry in Medicine, 1971, 2(1), 23-30.

The authors studied 28 children with ventricular septal defects (VSD). One half of the group had a surgical procedure for correction of the defect. Variables focused upon were intellectual functioning, emotional disturbance, and alteration of body image. Findings suggest that operated children do demonstrate significantly more impairment of intellectual functioning. No significant differences were found for the other variables although VSD children were found to be more similar emotionally to children in a psychiatric clinic than to a control group.

37. Auestad, A. M., & Naevested, M. Comparison of the therapeutic approaches to two children suffering from the aftereffects of physical illness and hospitalization. International Journal of Child Psychotherapy, 1973, 2(3), 345-364.

The authors present the case histories of two preschool children who required psychiatric help after experiencing physical illness and hospitalization. The differences in the personalities and families of the children and the resulting varying approaches to treatment and prognoses are described. The advantages of the parents' close cooperation and especially of the mother's presence during therapy are discussed.

38. Aufhauser, T. R. Child in the hospital. AORN, 1971, 13(5), 75-78.

For a long time efforts have been exerted to make hospitalization more tolerable for children. Changes in hospital environments and procedures are discussed, and the role of the nurse in dealing with the young child and his parents is examined.

39. Axelrod, B. H. Mental health considerations in the pediatric emergency room. Journal of Pediatric Psychology, 1976, 1(4), 14-17.

The emergency room setting provides an almost unending number of opportunities for psycho-social intervention, and yet this area of patient contact has been for the most part sorely neglected in most training programs throughout the United States. The purpose of this paper is to share the experience of the emergency room setting from the persepective both of the house officers and supportive staff who work there and of the families and children who must seek care under the most adverse conditions and finally to provide some suggestions for intervention which can be made regardless of professional discipline.

40. Ayer, A. H. Is partnership with parents really possible? MCN: American Journal of Maternal Child Nursing, 1978, 3(2), 107-110.

It is paradoxical that even in the most progressive institutions, where recognition of the need for primary providers of health care has led to the establishment of family practice clinics and primary nursing, the parents' primary role in the health care of their children often receives less than adequate encouragement. The author feels that there are several common reasons for this deficiency: (1) the structure of the unit is inadequate; (2) therapeutic considerations--parents are not trained personnel; (3) parents' participation might affect the level of staffing; and (4) nurses have nurturing needs that the parents may fulfill instead of them. The author addresses each of these points and outlines suggestions for how parents and staff can be better integrated in the treatment of hospitalized children.

41. Azarnoff, P. A play program in a pediatric clinic. Children, 1970, 17(6), 218-221.

Today many hospitals in this country provide play programs for hospitalized children as an important part of medical treatment. However, only a few pediatric outpatient clinics in the United States provide any activity programs for children and very few of these are conducted by paid staff members. The experience of the child activities program at the outpatient pediatric clinic of the University of California at Los Angeles is described to illustrate some of the important benefits that such a program can provide. With a clinic staff interested in the psychology of illness and crisis, with administrators willing to provide the necessary salaries, space, and budget, and with a volunteer program available to recruit, screen, and continuously train volunteers to help, a child activities program can show its worth.

42. Azarnoff, P. Mediating the trauma of serious illness and hospitalization in childhood. Children Today, 1974, 3(4), 12-17.

This article describes an Open Playroom at the University of California, Los Angeles, hospital and pediatric clinic in which play situations can occur naturally and spontaneously. When children become absorbed in play and informational sessions, they become more relaxed and less fearful. They are usually better able to cope with their concerns involving the equipment, procedures and people in the medical setting. Thus, in addition to their physical health, the children's emotional life is also favorably affected.

43. Azarnoff, P. Centers of learning in a pediatric clinic playroom. Journal of the Association for the Care of Children in Hospitals, 1975, 4(1), 33-38.

This article describes a number of different play opportunities which can better help the child to understand and cope with illness and hospitalization. A variety of materials are outlined and some case material presented to illustrate their application. In playgroups offering this variety of unrestricted opportunities for dramatic play, use of plastic and graphic materials, growing plants and animals, and interaction with the staff, the children can begin to objectify their private world and feelings into play situations, and by externalizing they are better able to alter, revise and deal with them. They can then feel more assured, cared for, and informed.

44. Azarnoff, P. The care of children in hospitals: An overview. Journal of Pediatric Psychology, 1976, 1(4), 5-6.

This article discusses innovations in child care and concludes that the past decade has brought a more integrated approach to dealing with children in hospitals including child life activities with opportunities for play, the preparation of children prior to events and the involvement of parents in their children's care. Research on hospitalization and children has grown, the available literature increasing from two to 500 in the last 40 years.

45. Azarnoff, P. Hospitalized children: How you can lessen the emotional impact. Resident and Staff Physician, 1976, May, 152-156.

This article points out that there are many ways for an individual physician to take first steps leading to the establishment of a child-life philosophy, or to have a smaller-scale play program for his pediatric patients. Some of these steps include: (1) Encourage parents of your patients to visit during mealtimes to feed their children or to be company for them; (2) Establish a temporary place for several children to sit together at meals; (3) Provide opportunities for parents to discuss with the dietician, or to write down the child's likes and dislikes in food; (4) Permit parents to bring some food to children on regular diets, as long as they tell the nurse; (5) Encourage children to bring to the hospital their favorite object, in order to have something in the environment that is familiar to him; (6) Discourage nurses from trying to break the child's habit of finger-sucking at this time of increased anxiety, no matter what the child's age; (7) If the child is used to falling asleep with a bottle, continue this practice during hospitalization if his condition permits; (8) Avoid middle-of-the-night procedures whenever possible. The author also discusses principles important to the nursing staff and additional points relevant to parents.

46. Azarnoff, P., & Flegal, S. A pediatric play program: Developing a therapeutic play program for children in medical settings. Springfield, Illinois: Charles C. Thomas, 1975.

This book tells how to set up a therapeutic play program for children in hospitals and clinics. Children in the medical milieu not only have the same developmental requirements which they had before they entered the hospital or clinic, but they also have new needs, having to adjust and adapt to difficulties never before encountered. With the necessary materials, space to play and with specially trained people, children can be helped to cope successfully with these difficulties and to master them, coming out of the experience stronger than before. Attention is given to typical low budgets and minimal staffing.

47. Bach, W. G. Teen-age patients. Hospitals, 1970, 44(2), 51-53.

Adolescent behavior should be examined within the context of development. The adolescent in a general hospital has specific needs in the areas of medicine, nursing, and hospital administration. Creating an adolescent unit undoubtedly increases the cost of structure, programming, and staff. However, if we truly wish to upgrade patient care, we no longer can be satisfied to treat adolescents in either pediatric or adult wards. An adolescent is not a child, though he periodically displays childish behavior. Nor is he an adult, even though he sometimes is more mature than the so-called adult patient. The adolescent is a very real person with special problems and needs--and worthy of our best understanding.

48. Barnes, C. M., Kenney, F. M., Call, T., & Reinhart, J. B. Measurement in management of anxiety in children for open heart surgery. <u>Pediatrics</u>, 1972, <u>49</u>(2), 250-259.

A study of neuro-endocrine and behavioral response to psychological stress of 11 children having heart surgery was initiated. An attempt was made to learn if more overtly anxious children would respond differently during hospitalization and surgery than those who appeared to have better emotional control. Assessment of anxiety in affect and function was made by a child psychiatrist and a pediatric nurse specialist during the hospitalization and at outpatient follow-up. Twenty-four-hour urine collections were made after suture removal and pre- and post-discharge and analyzed for 17-hydroxycosteroids by a modification of the method of Porter and Silber. In terms of emotional stimulation of the adrenocortical axis, the days before surgery and of return from intensive care were the most stressful of the days studied. The mean value on the day before surgery was significantly greater than that on the day before discharge. Values for the day before and after suture removal were also elevated in comparison with the day before discharge. Hospitalization was seen as stressful in terms of the parameter studied with the mean of all inpatient values including the day of discharge being approximately double that obtained by pooling all outpatient determinations. Surprising to the researchers was the fact that no difference was found between values for overtly excessively anxious children versus their less anxious counterparts on specific days, or when pooled in-hospital values were contrasted. The degree of elevation of 17-OHCS was related to the situation. No correlation between the estimate of anxiety and 17-OHCS levels was found. It is suggested that prognosis is greatly related to the coping capacity of a child and his family to stress; that prognoses can be predicted if adequate assessments can be made; and that as more precise methods for evaluation of the neuro-endocrine response become available it will be useful to employ them to explore the complicated relationship between the central nervous system and the endocrine organs in relation to children under stress.

49. Barnes, C. M. Levels of consciousness indicated by responses of children to phenomena in the intensive care unit. Maternal-Child Nursing Journal, 1975, 4(4, Monograph #4), 215-285.

The author studied school-age children's perceptions of phenomena and levels of consciousness in the Intensive Care Unit (ICU). Subjects were seven girls and six boys, hospitalized for heart surgery. Data were observations of the children, their drawings of the ICU, interviews, family relationships and dynamics, and pertinent medical histories. Data were analyzed in terms of categories of phenomena and levels of consciousness. Of the total responses, over half were classified as alert responses, and one-third as distorted. Most responses were to treatment and procedures. It was concluded that the children were very alert to ICU phenomena, but there was a high frequency of distortion. Children who had had deaths of relatives and other emotional experiences remembered them in the ICU.

50. Barnes, C. M. School-age children's recall of the intensive care unit. ANA clinical sessions, San Francisco, 1974. New York: Appleton-Century Crofts, 1975, 73-91.

A view of the intensive care unit by children who had heart surgery is presented here through observations, drawings, and interviews. General impressions and more specific responses were abstracted from data collected over a three-month period. The thirteen children ranged in age from six to sixteen years; there were ten boys and three girls. School age children responded to their experiences in the intensive care unit with negative impressions. The children vividly reported their memories of the nighttime. Most proclaimed that they could not sleep. Many said there were no nurses and doctors in the nighttime.

51. Barowsky, E. I. Young children's perceptions and reactions to hospitalization. In E. Gellert (Ed.), Psychosocial aspects of pediatric care. New York: Grune & Stratton, 1978, 37-49.

Adjustment to the exigencies of life is a developmental process, with the individual's abilities to cope predicated upon the previous establishment of healthy experiences and relationships. Hospitalization, which requires separation as well as adjustment to potentially threatening events, is one of these exigencies. Preparation, support, and protection from physical and psychological pain, while meeting the developing individual's daily needs, are indeed important; however, they cannot forestall or thwart anxieties which occur naturally. Recognition of these factors which contribute to maladjustment is essential in that their minimization will help the child to cope with new and often frightening experiences.

52. Bassett, J. A. There's a tavern in the playroom. Journal of the Association for the Care of Children in Hospitals, 1978, 6(3), 11-14.

This article discusses the use of music in a pediatric hospital's play room. The author discusses how to use homemade music and how to integrate puppets and theater in a play room program. Specific types of songs and puppet shows are presented as suggestions.

53. Battle, C. U. Chronic physical disease: Behavioral aspects. Pediatric Clinics of North America, 1975, 22(3), 525-531.

Being chronically ill is vastly different from being acutely ill. It stresses and drains the child and every family member over an indefinite period of time. Children with chronic physical disease are invariably depressed, with subtle or obvious signs of sadness. Moreover, having a chronic physical disease undermines the child's self-image, and ultimately his self-esteem. A handicapped child engenders a handicapped family, almost a universal phenomenon. This article discusses the pediatrician's goal in helping the family achieve the best adjustment possible in their particular circumstances. Additionally, the physician's role in assisting the family of the child with a fatal illness is outlined, and the significance of chronic hospitalization is examined.

54. Baxter, P. Frustration felt by a mother and her child during the child's hospitalization. MCN: American Journal of Maternal Child Nursing, 1976, 1(3), 159-161.

This article describes the experience of a nurse whose infant daughter was admitted to hospital. The mother-nurse observed many ways in which hospital personnel could ease the pain, uncertainty, and helplessness of patients and their families. After the experience, the author was determined to apply her new understanding to her profession as a nurse instructor.

55. Beardslee, C. The development of a trusting relationship in a two year old. Maternal-Child Nursing Journal, 1972, 1(3), 251-258.

This report describes the efforts made by a hospital nurse to persuade a two-year-old adopted boy to trust her. The subject was hospitalized for rectal bleeding and could not bear to be separated from his foster mother. Treatment involved playing games with a disappearing and reappearing theme. The first indication of trust occurred on the third day of contact when the boy learned to rely on the sameness of outer providers.

56. Beardslee, C. Factors which influence the sleep-wakefulness pattern of young, hospitalized children at nap time (Doctoral dissertation, University of Pittsburgh, 1974). Dissertation Abstracts International, 1974, 35(1-B), 345.

The problem of this study was to determine what variations in the immediate environment, level of malaise and stressful experiences of hospitalized, preschool children affected the onset, duration, and disruption of sleep during the scheduled daily nap time. Twenty-four children, two to five years of age, who were hospitalized for medical and surgical problems comprised the study sample. Each child was observed for four to six consecutive days. It was found that: (1) there was a tendency for both the interval of wakefulness and the duration of sleep to be longer on days when overt signs of malaise were lacking than when such signs were present; (2) the incidence of short intervals of wakefulness and long intervals of sleep was greatest on days when there was a low prevalence of stimuli occasioned by ongoing ward activities unrelated to the observed child; (3) the incidence of prolonged wakefulness was somewhat greater on days when stressful happenings occurred than when they did not; (4) sleep disruptions occurred in response to stimuli occasioned by on-going ward activities, activities of staff members which entailed physical contact with the child, and bodily discomfort; (5) the incidence of persisting wakefulness subsequent to disruption was higher than that of sleep resumption. On fifty-three of the eighty-nine sleep days, the scheduled nap time was not long enough to permit the children to complete their nap prior to the time the normal ward activities were resumed.

57. Beardslee, C. The sleep-wakefulness pattern of young hospitalized children during nap time. Maternal-Child Nursing Journal, 1976, 5(1), 15-24.

The author observed 24 hospitalized children two to five years old for four to six days each, beginning at lunch time and continuing through the end of the scheduled nap time. The children were in 1-, 2-, or multiple-bed rooms located for the most part on a heavily traveled corridor of the hospital. Results describe the duration of presleep, sleep, and sleep disruptions. Children slept for at least a short interval on 89 of the total 125 observation days. Mean duration of sleep was 41 minutes. Sleep duration appeared affected by the prevalence of ward activity unrelated to the observed child. The presence of staff members in the child's room appeared to have little effect on sleep unless there was direct physical contact. Stimuli contributing to sleep disruption are described, with their apparent effects.

Apparent separation anxiety interfered with sleep for children who were moved to different rooms immediately before scheduled nap time. Interference with sleep caused by external stimuli was higher when the body's need for sleep was reduced. It is suggested that hospital routines be adjusted so as to avoid high levels of environmental stimuli during scheduled nap time.

58. Beardslee, C., & Sperhac, A. Reaction formation in a pre-adolescent girl. Maternal-Child Nursing Journal, 1978, _7_(1), 31-40.

This article presents a case study of Sarah, an eleven year old girl, who entered the hospital with the chief complaint of lower abdominal cramps which had reportedly been experienced, on an intermittent but monthly basis, for a period of several months. Surgical exploration revealed that Sarah had an ovarian cyst and a vagina which ended blindly, rather than the suspected hematocolpos. Sarah was hospitalized a total of nineteen days--four days for diagnostic workup and fifteen days for sugical remediation and recuperation. During the hospitalization period there were many instances when Sarah's behavior was strongly suggestive of reaction formation. The behaviors in question were observed to occur at times when Sarah was exposed to olfactory and visual stimuli which were suggestive of uncontrolled discharges from the body. This article details Sarah's history, her symptoms, and defense mechanisms.

59. Beatty, A. Symposium on family-centered care in a pediatric setting: Foreword. Nursing Clinics of North America, 1972, _7_(1), 1-3.

It is the aim of this symposium to provide the reader with a well rounded picture of the important concept of family-centered care. Information from the behavioral sciences as well as nursing has been included. Emphasis has been placed on the treatment and care of the pediatric patient as a member of a particular family unit. The nature of the family unit itself has been looked at--its structure, its function in society, and the disruptive effects of illness on its members. Some of the major problems of meeting the basic human needs of patients have been examined, the role of the nurse has been discussed, and the collaborative role of nurses and other allied health personnel both in the hospital and in the community are outlined.

60. Beavers, B. C. An exploratory study of the psychological sequelae of surgery and hospitalization in male children (Doctoral dissertation, University of Southern California, 1974). Dissertation Abstracts International, 1974, 34(10-B), 5160.

The purpose of the study was to make a follow-up investigation of children who have had surgery for esophageal atresia and to explore the effects of such surgery and hospitalization on personality development. The main focus of the investigation was a study of the effects of prolonged hospitalization and traumatic surgical procedures on subsequent personality development. The present study is an exploratory investigation of whether the psychodynamic patterns of children born with this congenital anomaly are significantly different from those of children who have always been well, as defined by the norms of the instruments used. Assessment of subjects was made with regard to the following dimensions: general intellectual functioning, academic achievement, oral needs, ego ideal, self-concept, anxiety, and dependence proneness.

61. Becker, R. D. Therapeutic approaches to psychopathological reactions to hospitalization. International Journal of Child Psychotherapy, 1972, 1(2), 65-97.

A selective review of the recent clinical, psychoanalytic, and research literature on the psychopathological reactions of children to illness, surgery, or hospitalization is presented. A critical examination of an ostensibly "therapeutic" procedure, involving the use of puppets and dolls in "surgical play," is reconsidered and given close review. The notion that children invariably perceive their participation in these, sometimes "aggressive" and "mutilative," play activities as anxiety-reducing experiences is systematically challenged. Clinical evidence is presented to demonstrate that the indiscriminate use of these procedures may, in fact, have a paradoxically countertherapeutic effect on some children. An alternate clinical model for direct psychotherapeutic presurgical and postsurgical intervention, using the Mutual Storytelling Technique devised by Gardner (1971), is examined. Its clinical usefulness as a principal method of therapeutic communication with the hospitalized child is advanced.

62. Becker, R. D. Recent developments in child psychiatry--clinical paediatrics liaison consultation: (I) The restrictive emotional and cognitive environment reconsidered: A redefinition of the concept of therapeutic restraint. Israeli Annals of Psychiatry and Related Disciplines, 1975, 13(3), 239-258.

A selective review of the historical as well as the recent contemporary clinical, psychoanalytic and animal research literature on the subject of inadvertent psychopathological reactions of neonates, infants and children to illness-related cognitively-altered sensory, motor or physical environments in hospital, is presented. A critical reexamination of the concept of "therapeutic restraint" is systematically advanced and individual child-patient case histories are included documenting the author's contention that the new medical, orthopaedic and surgical advances attained and achieved in recent years are not without their attendent ubiquitous psychological liabilities. The psychic trauma of hospitalization with its too frequent disregard for the unarticulated fears and quiet anxieties of young children are discussed. Some straight-forward psycho-therapeutic guidelines are laid down with the hope that an informed and new approach will assist in the prevention of a host of otherwise predictably psychologically upsetting experiences for infants, children and indeed parents coming to hospital for reason of diagnostic assessment treatment of illness or operation.

63. Becker, R. D. Children in the hospital. Israeli Annals of Psychiatry and Related Disciplines, 1976, 14(3), 240-265.

This article discusses the emotional, affective, and

psychological responses of children (and their parents) to illness-related insulting experiences occurring in the hospital. Pediatric emotional response to hospitalization, surgical invasion, familial separation, assignment to an intensive care unit or to physical restraint are explored along with pediatric emotional and psychological response to upsetting diagnostic and medical intervention. Topics covered include radical surgical assault on the body image, post-surgical depressive reactions, and children's responses to therapeutic amputation, anesthesia, intractable pain, loss of control, protracted convalescence, and death. Psychotherapeutic guidelines for behavioral management of the acutely anxious child in biological or surgical crises are suggested along with specific indications for clinical psychiatric or psychological referral.

64. Bell, A. N. Psychological preparation of child contributes to success of surgery. Hospital Topics, 1971, 49(6), 78-79.

Preoperative preparation of children and their parents contributes as much to the success of surgery as technical skills of nurses, surgeons and anesthesiologists. It is true that a child can be prepared pharmacologically, but at Children's Hospital in Dallas, Texas, it is believed that psychological preparation is safer and returns the child to a more normal state of mind more rapidly. This article discusses various ways in which medical staff can prepare children for surgery.

65. Bell, G. J. Moths and butterflies. Pediatric Nursing, 1976, 2 (3), 36-41.

This article discusses the case history of a child who spent twelve of his first fifteen months of life in a hospital. The author and mother describes some of the common problems that parents of such children must face and discusses how nurses can minimize the deleterious effects of hospitalization on the family unit.

66. Bell, J. E., & Bell, E. A. Family participation in hospital care for children. Children, 1970, 17(4), 154-157.

During the middle part of the 1960's the authors of this article visited about 150 medical facilities in what are known as "developing countries" in Africa and Asia to study the part played by the patient's family in care in the hospital. They found members of the patients' families in almost all hospitals. To understand why relatives come or do not come to the hospital, it is necessary to look at the child, his family, the community from which the child comes, the hospital and its staff, and the complex interrelationships among them. In this report, observations are restricted to situations in which the patients were children. The authors conclude that participation of the family in hospital care is not an exotic curiosity, but a natural expression of family conviction strongly adhered to in three-fourths of the world. The practice is followed because it is a humane response to the rights of children. It is their belief that access to the best in health care is a right for all the children in the United States, and that family access to children in hospitals is equally a right.

67. Belmont, H. S. Hospitalization and its effects on the total child. Clinical Pediatrics, 1970, 9, 472-483.

Every child psychiatrist in his daily work draws on a multiplicity of resources from his diagnostic experiences. As this transcript of a lecture to resident psychiatrists points out, any thorough understanding of the effects of physical illness and hospitalization upon a child calls for a synthesis of knowledge concerning genetic, maturational and developmental factors as well as insights into the psychodynamics of conflict.

68. Bernstein, D. M. After transplantation--the child's emotional reactions. American Journal of Psychiatry, 1971, 127(9), 1189-1193.

This study examined the emotional responses and adaptation of 36 children who had received renal transplants.

They were examined immediately following their hospital discharge and upon return visits to a post transplant clinic up to six years later. Of the 32 children who survived, four showed significant emotional reactions. One adolescent, hospitalized for kidney rejection, manifested a moderate depressive reaction. Two adolescent boys displayed counterphobic reaction, with risk-taking behavior. One adolescent girl manifested phobias, with school refusal. The others were all in school full time and without major emotional problems. The author stresses the need for alertness on the part of the nephrologist, surgeon, and psychiatrist in dealing with emotional problems of child transplant patients.

69. Beuf, A. H. Biting off the bracelet: A study of children in hospitals. Philadelphia: University of Pennsylvania Press, 1979.

The observations that underlie this book were carried out by participant observation in two hospitals. In "County Hospital," where observations were carried out in 1971 and 1972, the researcher also acted as a visitor to ill children. At "Metropolis," observations were carried out in the admissions area, the waiting rooms, and on the floors, where the researcher acted as a worker with the play-therapists and as a visitor. The book is about the social situation of the hospitalized child in twentieth-century America. It contends that the children's hospital has many of the characteristics of depersonalization and enforced helplessness that are associated with other "total institutions" in our society. It also examines the interpersonal approaches employed by staff and patients in dealing with the tensions created by the reality of the total institution on the one hand, and the more idealistic goals of the children's hospital on the other. Some measures are suggested that might improve this situation.

70. Bezzeg, B. D. Please, don't run away. Journal of the Association for the Care of Children in Hospitals, 1975, 3(4), 9-13.

The creation of a "health-oriented" approach to children and their families in what has long been a "pathology-oriented" system is a remarkable accomplishment for which the Child Care in Hospital movement deserves much credit. Examination of some of the elements of its construction provides clues for continuing effort to support the child and his family by the health care institution, and to research the effects of such programs. The significant areas in which the Child Care in Hospitals movement has created change are in: (1) the administrative policies of institutions providing health services for children; (2) the establishment of child-centered programs and staff in health care settings; (3) the inclusion of child developmental needs as a legitimate area of education for health care personnel; and (4) innovative programming of preventive mental health for children as a part of health care services.

71. Billington, G. F. Play program reduces children's anxiety, speeds recoveries. Modern Hospital, 1972, 118(4), 90-92.

The child in the hospital is a stranger in a strange world. His loneliness and apprehension, besides affecting his mental state, can also impede his medical progress. Organized play can help effect a feeling of calm, relaxation and security, ease homesickness, relieve nervous tension, and serve as an outlet for constructive ideas and activities. As children become more relaxed, they make fewer demands on the nurses for attention and reassurance, and the entire pediatric unit takes on an atmosphere of controlled care. This article describes the development and implementation of a play program undertaken at Elizabeth General Hospital and Dispensary in New Jersey.

72. Birchfield, M. E. Nursing care for hospitalized children based on different stages of illness. MCN: American Journal of Maternal Child Nursing, 1981, 6(1), 46-51.

While working in a 24-bed pediatric unit of a general midwestern hospital the author developed an illness continuum approach that integrates knowledge of the stages of illness with nursing care interventions. The four identified stages of illness include: (1)

non-acute; (2) acute; (3) post-acute; and (4) terminal. The author discusses age appropriate interventions helpful to the hospitalized child at each point along this continuum.

73. Blos, P., Jr. Children think about illness: Their concepts and beliefs. In E. Gellert (Ed.), Psychosocial aspects of pediatric care. New York: Grune & Stratton, 1978, 1-18.

Basically, children are researchers. This raging curiosity includes their own bodies, how they function, and why things go wrong, as they invariably do. For every question there must be an answer which the child obtains by a mixture of observation, thought, fantasy, previous experience, and prior explanation. But the effectiveness of this research is limited by intruded affect, and the child's current level of cognitive function, need for defense, and opportunities for observation. This chapter reviews some of the studies that have explored children's ideas, concepts, and understanding of matters pertaining to their body's health, illness, treatment and death. It then discusses the applicability of this material to clinical work with children.

74. Blumberg, M. L. Depression in children on a general pediatric service. American Journal of Psychotherapy, 1978, 32(1), 20-32.

Masked depression in the hospitalized child is precipitated by maternal separation and anxiety aggravated by environmental, somatic, and existing personality factors. Age, stage of ego development, and comprehension are important influences. Psychiatrically oriented as well as somatically indicated therapy is essential for a favorable outcome. Parents require supportive consideration also.

75. Bowden, M. S. How we did it: Family centered care in a large community hospital. Journal of the Association for the Care of Children in Hospitals, 1979, 8(1), 14-17.

This article outlines the implementation of family centered care through the Department of Maternal Child Nursing at the Tucson Medical Center. The author discusses important program changes made in each of four areas: Pediatrics, Nurseries, Maternity, and Labor and Delivery. Specific suggestions for how other children's hospitals might benefit are presented.

76. Bradley, M. Parent-patient-doctor relationships in a surgical children's ward in a large teaching hospital. Proceedings of the Royal Society of Medicine, 1972, 65(4), 336-338.

Good parent-child-staff relationships are essential in any children's ward for the physical and psychological well-being of the child, for good rapport and exchange of information at all levels, for effective functioning of the ward staff as a team, and for the care of the child in a loving, trusting environment where he is treated as an individual and a member of his family. This article discusses the problems that can arise when a child is in hospital, first in relation to the individuals concerned, and secondly in connection with particular circumstances.

77. Brandt, P. A., Smith, M. E., Ashburn, S. S., & Graves, J. IM injections in children. American Journal of Nursing, 1972, 72(8), 1402-1406.

Intramuscular injection administration is one procedure that involves predictable pain. How a child responds to the injection depends, in part, on his developmental age and his previous experience. Children show a wide range of reactions and coping mechanisms when confronted with this form of medicinal administration. As she gives an injection, the nurse's approach must vary according to her assessment of the child's level of biophysical and psychosocial development. The nurse's approach, therefore, will not only vary with each child but will also vary, to a certain degree, with the same child each time she must give the child an injection. This article discusses some age-related factors helpful in understanding the child's response to injections.

78. Brazelton, T. B. The emotional needs of children in health care settings. Clinical Proceedings of the Children's Hospital National Medical Center, 1976, 32(8), 157-166.

This article discusses some of the things that could aid health care professionals in terms of setting up a different model of looking beyond people's defenses, beyond the illness or the symptom they present with, to a model of how they have coped and what is available to work with that will help them deal with illness and hospitalization. The failure-to-thrive syndrome in hospitalized children is discussed within the framework of Bowlby's three stages of separation: protest, despair and detachment. The role of parents of the hospitalized child is examined, and suggestions for the preparation of children for hospitalization are presented.

79. Brazelton, T. B. Listening to toddlers. Journal of the Association for the Care of Children in Hospitals, 1976, 4(3), 17-20.

Implicit in the theme of this paper is the reminder that parents and the children themselves are part of the medical team. Unless physicians listen, they may indeed miss the important cues which can tell them what it is they have available to them in the way of strengths, of past experiences, of needs to help them cope with the immediate experiences of being ill, being separated, hospitalized in unnatural conditions, and of being hurt and frightened. Implicit in the medical model are several mechanisms which may well interfere with the capacity to listen. First we are taught to play "God"; we must be the experts, we must be in control, we must be right, or our very roles are endangered. Second, we are taught to look for pathology. There is no premium on looking for the strengths of a child or his parents. And third, most of us are not trained for or ready for therapeutic relationships with our patients. The author makes a plea for a realization that if we are willing to look and listen to people, we are in a position to make a real transference relationship within which we can have a very different diagnostic and therapeutic effect.

80. Brink, P. J. Critique of "Passage through hospitalization of severely burned, isolated school-age children." Communicating Nursing Research, 1975, 7, 198-203.

This article presents a critique of a study concerned with the identification of patterns and sequence of behavior in severely burned, isolated children age six to ten years during initial hospitalization and immediately upon return home. The emphasis of the critique is upon the analysis of data, but the research narrative itself as it conforms to the mandates of science is reviewed, as well.

81. Brooks, M. M. Why play in the hospital? Nursing Clinics of North America, 1970, 5(3), 431-441.

Since World War II, largely because of increasing understanding of child development, there has been a change of focus from disease-oriented to patient-oriented pediatric care. The total climate of the pediatric unit or pediatric hospital has changed and is changing as those responsible for the child in the hospital begin to recognize his needs and try to meet them. There is much still to be learned, especially about the care of infants, and much that is already known that must be put into practice. In this discussion the authors examine the total hospital environment in order to see how it meets the needs of young children, with special reference to the way in which these needs can be served through an organized program of constructive play activities carried out under professional supervision.

82. Brooks, M. M. Programmed play complements care. Hospitals, 1973, 47(15), 78-87.

Separation from familiar surroundings, from home, and from family naturally arouses a child's anxiety, especially during the preschool years. At the Children's Hospital, Philadelphia, a program of appropriate-age activities provides constructive outlets for such apprehension and prevents serious and long-lasting psychological problems that might accrue. Parental anxiety is examined.

83. Brooks, M. M. Improving care for the hospitalised child: A universal need. Australasian Nurses Journal, 1976, 5, 51-53.

This article presents a summary of the efforts of individuals and organizations to make hospitalization a better experience for children and their families. The author refers to the work of many professionals who contributed to the development of an increased awareness and interest in the welfare of children in hospitals. The main portion of the article deals with the Association for the Care of Children in Hospitals, a multidisciplinary organization formed for the purpose of promoting and fostering the well-being of children in health care settings. The article discusses the growth and scope of the association. Emphasis is placed on educational programs, the ACCH Journal, and the need for research to promote further change.

84. Brown, B. Beyond separation: Some new evidence on the impact of brief hospitalization on young children. In D. Hall and M. Stacy (Eds.), Beyond separation: Further studies of children in hospital. London: Routledge & Kegan Paul, Ltd., 1979, 18-53.

This chapter explores the theoretical background and assumptions of much of the earlier work on children in hospital, which has been dominated by concerns with deprivation and maternal separation. These concepts are interpreted as aspects of a more general balance theory, which sees attachment behavior in children as an evolutionary response to threat and separation from mother. Using this perspective, the author reviews a number of other hospital studies and shows that although the observations of disturbance in hospital, and in particular the phases of disturbance reported by Robertson and Bowlby, are explicable in terms of this model, it is less easy to explain variations in the severity of the outcome of a stay in hospital for different children. He concludes that the emphasis on discontinuity which is found in balance theory must be expanded from a purely psychological orientation to include a sociological component. Here the meaning of discontinuity would include the disruptions to the social life of the child occasioned by hospital treatment.

85. Brown, M. J. Preadmission orientation for children and parents. Canadian Nurse, 1971, 66, 29-31.

This article describes a preadmission orientation program for children at the Royal Alexandra Hospital, Edmonton, Alberta, which is an attempt to reduce anxiety in children about to be admitted to hospital for elective surgery. Although there have been no official studies to measure the effectiveness of this program, the nursing staff have noted a difference in the attitudes of children who have participated in their orientation program. Anesthesiologists at the hospital have stated that they too can identify those children who have been prepared for hospitalization through the orientation program. This program seems to have the greatest effect on children between four and six years of age. The results of this kind of program indicate the desirability of some form of pre-hospitalization orientation. Factors to be considered in determining content and presentation of the orientation programs are: (1) the child's age; (2) time of preparation; (3) information pertinent for parents; and (4) information necessary for the child. More research is required to determine the effectiveness of existing programs and to investigate means of improving them. A need exists for educative measures that can reduce the psychological stress of hospitalization for the child.

86. Brown, V. Providing a safe environment for children. MCN: American Journal of Maternal Child Nursing, 1978, 3(1), 53-55.

This article discusses federal requirements for full-sized baby cribs as a means of ensuring safe environments for hospitalized children. Safety requirements for children's toys are also outlined with suggestions for toy selection by hospital nursing staffs. The author hopes that review of such safety principles will help reduce the estimated 50,000 child crib injuries and the 700,000 toy-related child injuries which occur each year.

87. Bruce, T. J. R. Very ill children. Developmental Medicine and Child Neurology, 1974, 16(5), 675-677.

Doctors, nurses, and intensive care units are frightening to a baby or child who is admitted to the hospital. This article discusses what can be done to help children and families in intensive care units. Older children can be talked--and listened--to about their difficulties, and special techniques can be used to help them get things clear. But for both older and younger children, and for babies, the most important thing that can be done is to keep them in touch with their families--particularly with their mothers. Suggestions are made for group meetings of all health care professionals who attend a child hospitalized in an intensive care unit.

88. Burgdorf, M. M. Coping behaviors of a school age child hospitalized with burns. Maternal-Child Nursing Journal, 1978, 7(1), 11-19.

This paper reports a study of one school-age child, Johnny, age seven and a half, who was hospitalized because of a burn injury. Excerpts from nursing process data are presented to depict some of the experiences that this child encountered in the hospital and his responses to them. The coping behaviors that the child demonstrated before and after surgery for skin grafts are described and compared.

89. Burr, S. Play for children in hospital. Nursing Times, 1977, March (ABPN Supplement), 5-6.

This article briefly discusses the usefulness of play for hospitalized children. The main emphasis of the report is to provide information regarding voluntary organizations particularly concerned with play for children in hospital. A list of books containing rhymes, stories, activities, etc. helpful in play therapy is also provided.

90. Burrows, S. Taking fear out of pediatric patients. Hospital Topics, 1974, 52, 1.

This short article describes a pre-hospitalization puppet program geared for pre-surgical children. The children are introduced to the hospital and hospital procedures through the use of puppets which were made to look like a doctor, nurse, boy and a girl. Children are given some idea of what to expect when they are admitted to the hospital, and the daily routine in pediatrics is discussed. Since children are given a chance to play-act hospital, surgery is made less traumatic through the pediatric play program. There is a "play suitcase" which contains a family of dolls, including a doctor and a nurse doll, and hospital related toys such as I.V.'s, syringes with needles, bandages, tongue blades and stethoscope. Children are encouraged to play with these and work out their feelings.

91 Butler, A., Chapman, J., & Stuible, M. Child's play is therapy. Canadian Nurse, 1975, 71(12), 35-37.

The authors show how the therapeutic use of play makes hospitalization easier and more pleasant for the pre-school child. A few simple toys or props and the presence of an attentive adult are all that are needed. Play can be a simple, effective way of helping the pre-school child to deal with the strange and sometimes painful hospital world and to master situations that might otherwise be overwhelming. This type of play can be incorporated easily into the nursing care plan and can become an essential aspect of the care of the hospitalized preschool child. The results are rewarding in terms of happier, less anxious children, parents, and nursing staff.

92. Byers, M. L. Play interviews with a five-year-old boy. Maternal-Child Nursing Journal, 1972, 1(2), 133-141.

It is well known that permanent alteration of body image and function presents long term and complex problems to children, their families, and health professionals. In many institutions, the trend is toward short term hospitalization. An attempt is made here to learn more about the problems and crises children encounter and try to master during brief stays in the hospital so that the nurse's helping role may be more clearly defined. In the normal course of family development, preschool age children are involved in a psychosocial developmental crisis. This crisis intensifies and becomes more complex when illness or accidental injury occurs. The child discussed in this paper was a five-and-a-half year old boy who was hospitalized for smoke inhalation and small second-degreee burns on both feet and on one hand. The themes present in the child's play activities are explored.

93. Calkin, J. D. Are hospitalized toddlers adapting to the experience as well as we think? MCN: American Journal of Maternal Child Nursing, 1979, 4(1), 18-23.

To assess the behavioral adjustment of the hospitalized toddler, the author has developed a five dimension scale based on the developmental framework of Erik Erikson. Although the scales have not been rigorously tested for reliability and validity, they have been used systematically by graduate students in pediatric nursing as well as by undergraduate students and registered nurses in two hospitals. The results were so encouraging that other nurses may wish to test the scales in their own settings, for they represent a fruitful approach to determining whether or not a toddler's behavior is adaptive. In addition, nurses may find the framework useful for developing similar instruments to use with younger or older people. Major areas of assessment in the scales include: (1) toileting; (2) eating; (3) resting and sleeping; (4) separation from and return to a familiar person; and (5) indications of independence or emotional dependence on adults.

94. Campbell, J. D. Illness is a point of view: The development of children's concepts of illness. Child Development, 1975, 46(1), 92-100.

To study development of concepts of illness 264 children (6 to 12-11) and their mothers were interviewed. Comparison of group profiles showed that the typical definition given by children was similar to that of mothers: those used by many mothers were often used by children; those rare in mothers' definitions infrequently occurred in children's. Yet comparison of mother-child pairs revealed that the illness concept of any specific child was not likely to resemble that of his parent. With increasing maturity, children defined illness more precisely and placed greater emphasis on the performance and psychosocial dispositional states. Age-linked intellectual development and health experiences as moderated by age contributed to more adult-like, qualitatively more sophisticated definitions of illness.

95. Campbell, J. D. The child in the sick role: Contributions of age, sex, parental status, and parental values. Journal of Health and Social Behavior, 1978, 19(1), 35-51.

Information from 264 children (short-term patients in a pediatric hospital) and their mothers was evaluated to study the process that shapes perspectives on illness behavior and the sick role. Children's reports of how they acted when ill--their emotionality, rejection of the sick role, and communication of sick-role identification--were clearly tied to their age and sex roles and were significantly related to parental socioeconomic status (SES) indicators as well. A "Spartan" orientation toward illness was characteristic of older children, boys, and children of parents with higher SES. In part, attributes of status made their contributions to children's sick-role appraisals indirectly: Maternal valuations of the child's self-direction and self-assertion (two general parental values that were themselves responsive to status) provided a link between the social structure and children's assessments of their actions when ill. The impact of these values occurs primarily in the later years of childhood.

96. Campbell, L. Special behavioral problems of the burned child. American Journal of Nursing, 1976, 76(2), 220-224.

Burned children of any age and their families face overwhelming stress. For a severely burned child, the healing process involves prolonged hospitalization that includes isolation, immobilization, repeated trips to the operating room, extreme pain and discomfort, disfigurement, and total dependence on many people who are, at first, strangers. Often these children and their families have lost one or more friends or relatives in the accident in which they were injured. Early treatment of children who are severely burned is described, and suggestions for helping the parents of these victims are given. In addition, steps which can be taken by nursing staff to aid the victims and their families are discussed. Included is a discussion of how nursing intervention can help the child deal with his damaged concept of self due to disfigurement.

97. Canright, P., & Campbell, M. J. Nursing care of the child and his family in the emergency department. Pediatric Nursing, 1977, 3 (4), 43-45.

Children fear the emergency room itself because the environment is different and the roles of significant others change. They know from experience that when they are hurt someone who loves them is usually there to fix the hurt with minimal amount of discomfort. The emergency room setting is very different from the above situation. To help establish a better relationship with the child, the nurse should try to get down on their level and communicate with them using language the child can understand. Most parents can help calm their child. They may be helpful to the nurse or physician in interpreting what is happening to the child because they know their child's usual responses. They can be reassuring and often help in treatment.

98. Carey, W. B., & Sibinga, M. S. Avoiding pediatric pathogenesis in the management of acute minor illness. Pediatrics, 1972, 49(4), 553-562.

The management of acute minor illnesses constitutes a major portion of a physician's work. The impact of such illness on the child's development and physician's positive or negative influence on the child's and the parents' emotional adjustment are considered here. Very few data are available in the literature. Suggestions for management and research are presented. Diagnosis and therapy of acute minor illness are far from uniform or agreed upon. Accurate diagnosis and reasonable treatment are the pediatrician's first responsibility. Over-, under-, and misdiagnosing and treating are to be avoided. Secondly, he should nurture the sick child by reducing stress and by promoting his adjustment to the illness situation. The child's emotional health suffers from the pediatrician's neglect, over-involvement with or mismanagement of his feelings during illness. Thirdly, the pediatrician should support the parents by helping them to deal with the specific illness and by promoting their capacity to cope with illness in general. If, instead, the pediatrician is overly dominant or submissive, neglectful or punitive in handling the parents' needs, they may become frightened, dependent, demanding, confused, or angry. Their feelings of incompetence in handling illnesses affect their general child-raising abilities.

99. Carter, M. D. Identification of behaviors displayed by children experiencing prolonged hospitalization. <u>International Journal of Nursing Studies</u>, 1973, <u>10</u>(2), 125-135.

The purpose of this study is to identify those behaviours displayed by children experiencing prolonged hospitalization, and to determine the way in which the child perceives himself in this situation. One eight year old boy was tested using the Devereux Child Behaviour Rating Scale. The results suggested that the child exhibited marked problems in eleven of the seventeen behaviour factors studied, including: (1) Distractibility; (2) Pathological use of senses; (3) Emotional detachment; (4) Social isolation; (5) Poor co-ordination and body tonus; (6) Messiness, sloppiness; (7) Inadequate need for independency; (8) Proneness to emotional upset; (9) Need for adult contact; (10) Inability to delay; and (11) Social aggression. The data, though limited to only one subject, would seem to imply that children, experiencing long-term hoppitalization, do exhibit behaviours which may indiate problem areas.

100. Cartier, T. M. Anal compulsive behaviors of one four-and-a-half year old hospitalized boy. Maternal-Child Nursing Journal, 1980, 9 (2), 117-126.

James, the subject of this paper, was a four and one-half year old white male who was admitted to the hospital for diagnostic workup of a malabsorption problem which he had had since birth. From the time he was eighteen months old, James had been on a gluten-free diet. According to his father, when James ate any food with even traces of gluten he would suffer violent spells of abdominal cramps and diarrhea. Medical testing indicated that there was no physical reason for these problems. This case study presentation discusses how James developed anal compulsive behaviors and how these were at times exacerbated by hospitalization. Treatment of his psychological problems is also described.

101. Caudle, P. R. K., & Potter, J. Characteristics of burned children and the after effects of the injury. British Journal of Plastic Surgery, 1970, 23(1), 63-65.

More children under the age of five years are recorded dying from thermal injuries than from any other cause except traffic accidents. It is therefore of interest to enquire into the characteristics of children suffering burns and into the after-effects in those who survive. This was the purpose of a small-scale survey relating to 119 children (below the age of 15) who were admitted to the plastic surgery wards of the Stockton-on-Tees Children's Hospital as a result of burns or scalds. Results indicated that the majority of mothers were well satisfied with the treatment and care their children had received in hospital. Just over half the mothers thought that their children had been affected at least temporarily by staying in hospital; 38 mentioned the child crying, fretting or being distressed either at visiting time or especially on admission to hospital. Many mothers mentioned symptoms of distress occurring within a few days or weeks of the child returning home such as over-eating, clinging, weeping, being very quiet, over-nervous, frightened or restless at night. There was no apparent relationship in this group between long-term symptoms as mentioned by the parents, and either the seriousness of the accident, as measured by the skin area affected, or the length of stay in hospital. The majority of the mothers did not think that the accident had affected their child's relationship with other children or their progress at school.

102. Chadwick, B. J., Pflederer, D., & Ray, M. A. Maintaining the hospitalized child's home ties. American Journal of Nursing, 1978, 78(8), 1360-1362.

Separation of parent and child may be inevitable during hospitalization, but it need not be a negative experience for either parent or child. Nurses can take concrete action to help the child maintain attachment relationships during this crisis situation. Such action begins with an assessment of the attachment interaction between child and parents as soon as the child is admitted to the hospital. Types of attachment behaviors the child displays toward his parents should be noted, and validation must be sought from the parents to check the accuracy of these observations and conclusions. Additionally, the nurse should find out whether or not the parents can remain with the child, visit periodically, or will not come again until discharge. Although a child may be very upset after a parent leaves, an approach which is honest and reassuring and lets the child know what to expect in terms of visitation, is psychologically better for the child than being dishonest.

103. Chaloner, L. Children and hospitals. Nursing Mirror, 1972, 134(2), 11-12.

This article describes the work of the National Association for the Welfare of Children in Hospitals. The main aspects of the study were to discover what happens to handicapped children physically and emotionally during their stay in hospital, then to plan and implement the changes found to be necessary and disseminate the findings. Obviously, the medical needs of individual children take priority, but the emphasis is on providing as normal a life for each child as his handicapping condition permits.

104. Chan, J. M. Child life therapists help humanize hospitalization. Hospitals, 1977, 51(21), 14, 16, 20.

The rationale for and the value of child life programs are being recognized by more and more hospitals. The programs in force today differ markedly in specific functions--providing school learning situations, recreation, play experiences, child advocacy, or any combination thereof--but share a common denominator in that they strive to make hospitalization less traumatic for children. One such program, staffed by four salaried child life therapists which has been in effect since 1974 at Doernbecher Memorial Hospital for Children at the University of Oregon Health Sciences Center in Portland, is described. An important aspect of this program is the training, in-service education, and supervision provided by the department of child psychiatry, which jointly sponsors the program with the department of pediatrics. Another aspect of the ongoing education of the child life therapist is the review and discussion of current literature on children and their care.

105. Clark, D. Parents' meetings in a pediatric unit: Helping parents cope with their child's hospitalization. Journal of the Association for the Care of Children in Hospitals, 1979, 8(2), 32-35.

This article discusses the use of parent meetings established at Sinai Hospital in Baltimore. The goals of these groups are: (1) to provide an opportunity to share and ventilate feelings in a group with other parents experiencing a similar situation; (2) to answer questions regarding policy, procedures, or concerns; and (3) to inform staff of problems that parents are experiencing so that appropriate intervention can occur. Major themes ussually emerging within the group include: (1) problems in communicating with the hospital staff; (2) concerns about the level of care provided by the nursing staff when the parents are not present; (3) guilt and anger over the child's illness; and (4) decisions about the amount of visitation and/or rooming in. These group meetings are viewed as helpful to both parents and staff as well as to the overall care of the hospitalized child.

106. Clatworthy, S. M. The effect of therapeutic play on the anxiety behaviors of hospitalized children (Doctoral dissertation, Boston University School of Education, 1978). Dissertation Abstracts International, 1978, 38(12-B), 6142.

This study investigated the effects of therapeutic play on 23 five to twelve year old hospitalized children. Hospitalized children's anxiety levels were obtained from the pre-, post-, and pre/post measurements of the Missouri Children's Picture Series. Baseline anxiety was measured with the Missouri Children's Behavior Checklist completed by the parents at the time of their children's admission. Current levels of the child's anxiety as perceived by their parents was collected at admission and discharge. Additional pre-, post-, and pre/post data were collected from the children, parents, and assigned nurses. Child and parent interviews, child drawings of the hospital and their diagnosis, and nurses' ratings of behavior, provided information regarding the child's demonstrated behaviors and projected feelings. Content analysis was applied to all additional data. Findings included an increase of anxiety, regression, withdrawal and docility on the part of the control children, whereas the experimental children maintained the same measured level of anxiety at both admission and discharge. The experimental children were reported by their parents and nurses to be active, engaged in social activities and verbally expressed their feelings regarding their hospital experience. The parents of both groups of children consistently rated their child as less anxious than did the children themselves.

107. Cleary, J. Demands and responses: The effects of the style of work allocation on the distribution of nursing attention. In D. Hall and M. Stacy (Eds.), Beyond separation: Further studies of children in hospital. London: Routledge & Kegan Paul, Ltd., 1979, 109-127.

This chapter considers the link between the attitudes, orientations and activities of nursing staff and the behavior of children in hospital. On the basis of hospital observations undertaken during a hospital Playleader research project, data was collated relating to staff-patient contact from three separate weeks of ward observation, from case studies of children in a pediatric ward and from diary records kept by observers. The author concludes that although it is possible to reduce the number of inpatient admissions among children, it seems likely that for most of those whose admission is inevitable, care will remain principally in the hands of the nursing staff. In order to lessen distress within hospital, to cut down the number of clinically unhelpful events and reduce undesirable behavioral sequelae, both short and long term, it is necessary to change the orientation and the organization of the work within the ward, so that it will provide a more satisfactory response to the needs of the child patient. This chapter provides further evidence for regarding children's disturbance in hospital as only one feature of a complex problem involving staff and patients in the treatment of illness.

108. Clegg, R. L. Effects of a child life program upon the anxiety levels of children hospitalized for major elective surgery (Doctoral dissertation, University of Maryland, 1972). Dissertation Abstracts International, 1973, 33(9-B), 4882.

The major purpose of this investigation was to determine the effects of a selected Child Life Program upon the anxiety levels of children hospitalized for major elective surgery. The subjects were twenty females and twenty males who ranged in age from six to nine years. The surgical techniques employed varied from a simple procedure to extensive surgical intervention. The procedure for collecting data consisted of administering the Palmar Sweat Print (PSP) during hospital admission and following the termination of the surgical procedure yet prior to entry into the Child Life Program. The PSP was also administered after 4, 8, 12, and 16 hours of exposure to the Child Life Program and upon hospital discharge. The findings of this study evidenced a significant reduction in the anxiety levels of the total group following 4 hours of exposure to the Child Life Program and upon discharge from the hospital. The female and male subjects evidenced a statistically significant reduction in anxiety during exposure to the Child Life Program. The effects of the Child Life Program on the anxiety levels of the female and male subjects were not significant according to age. The female subjects evidenced a significant decrease in the anxiety levels after 4 hours of exposure and upon discharge from the hospital according to social position.

The male subjects demonstrated no statistically significant decrease in anxiety levels according to social position.

109. Cline, F. W., & Rothenberg, M. B. Preparation of a child for major surgery. Journal of the American Academy of Child Psychiatry, 1974, 13(1), 78-94.

The present paper details the experience of Bobby, a seven-year-old middle-class, Caucasian boy, with open heart surgery. Many problems were present which portended a poor prognosis. The authors follow Bobby's treatment chronologically as it developed. Transcripts obtained from audio and video tape recordings made during interview and play sessions were subsequently used in supervision. During treatment, a number of transactional and technical problems unexpectedly developed. A discussion concerning these issues follows the case presentation. The various psychological problems attendant in Bobby's case are discussed and the techniques used in helping the child prepare for surgery are presented.

110. Clough, F. Staff ratings of children's behaviour in hospital: Comparability of factor structures. British Journal of Psychology, 1978, 69(1), 59-68.

Behavior ratings for 108 nine to fifteen year old female orthopedic inpatients were obtained concurrently from three independent groups of ward-staff observers. Ratings were factor analyzed both within observer groups, and across groups (using mean scale item scores), and factorial structures were analyzed for comparability. It was found that the independently derived group structures were highly similar, replicating a four-dimensional system common to a number of analyses in other social settings, and recently given prominence in a review by E. Howarth (1976). In particular, the separation of fearful from hostile emotional behaviors and from a neutral sociability dimension was predicted and confirmed. However, while correlations between matched factor loadings were generally high, those between matched factor scores were much lower. It is argued that the procedure of averaging judges' ratings prior to factor analysis is useful not only to increase reliability, but also to improve validity by extending the range of sampling across different role situations. The combined solution offers a more valid composite criterion of "characteristic ward behavior," having a high multiple correlation with the independently derived predictor group observations.

111. Clough, F. The validation of meaning in illness-treatment situations. In D. Hall and M. Stacey (Eds.), Beyond separation: Further studies of children in hospital. London: Routledge & Kegan Paul, Ltd., 1979, 54-81.

This chapter examines the possibility of mismatch between social and personal meanings and outcomes in terms of observed behavior as they relate to the hospitalized child. In order to explicate the model of meanings mediating between social background and observed behaviors, a study was made of 104 girls aged 9 to 16 years in the orthopedic wards of three hospitals. Using factor analysis, aspects of children's meaning systems were related with staff's assessment of their behavior to produce an empirical classification of distinct areas of concern identified with the home, the ward, illness and treatment. The types of relationship predicted by the model were found, and the analysis provides a better insight into the way in which disorders of meaning and disorders of behavior go together. Differences in educational level rather than age as such were related to differences in the organization of meaning held by younger and older children. The results are discussed in terms of a theory of discrepancy, where disruption of a system of meanings lead to anomie.

112. Coffey, H., & Koch, C. R. Psycho-social care of the paralyzed child: A technique in intensive care nursing. Pediatric Nursing, 1975, 1(5), 21-23.

To relieve the trauma of hospitalization, the Intensive Care staff at The Children's Hospital of Philadelphia has employed the use of a cassette recorder with an ear plug jack and a program of tapes personally designed to help treat young patients. The effectiveness of the technique was demonstrated in the case of a two and one half year old girl named Laurie, who was admitted to the hospital with a primary diagnosis of acute lymphoblastic leukemia. The use of this technique for paralyzed and/or critically ill children such as Laurie had four distinct advantages: (1) Familiar voices on a continuous basis, coupled with programmed silence for rest and tapes for recreation, reassured the child that she was in a safe environment; (2) Parental participation in the program contributed to the psychological well-being of the child and helped control the parents' anxiety as well as reinforce their roles as the child's principal guardians; (3) The tapes diminished the nursing staff's concerns about its inability to provide constant communication with the child; and (4) The technique minimized post-intensive care and/or post-hospitalization regression and ameliorated behavioral disturbances.

113. Colaianni, J. A. Parents care in intensive care. Pediatric Nursing, 1975, 1(2), 16-19.

An important aspect of the Pediatric Intensive Care Unit at Children's Hospital, Philadelphia, is the enormous amount of emphasis which is placed on establishing and maintaining a normal maternal/child relationship. Children's Hospital has 24 hour visiting for parents, but the ICU differs in having five minute visiting every two hours. As the patient's condition can accommodate more time with the family, the visiting time is increased. Care of the child is never interrupted by a parent's visit. A day's activities are planned for each child--a routine which must be accomplished for his physical and psychological care. The staff allows the mother to be with the child while treatment is being administered. She is told exactly what is being done or will be done and is given the option to stay or leave. She may be involved in the bathing, feeding, and mothering of her child. Nurses actually plot out what she can or cannot do while her child is in the intensive care unit. If it is rest period, whether the mother is there or not, the child is left undisturbed. They never forget the importance of the maternal/child relationship, although it must be altered in view of the child's condition.

114. Coleman, K. P. Preventing and reducing anxiety in pediatric surgical patients: An educational and direct treatment approach (Doctoral dissertation, Kent State University, 1975). Dissertation Abstracts International, 1976, 36(9-A), 5819.

A total of 80 boys and girls, ranging in age from eight to 11, were selected and assigned to one of four groups containing 20 children in each. Experimental group #1 consisted of children scheduled for tonsillectomies who had not been previously hospitalized, and who participated in the play therapy and orientation treatment, following hospital admission. Experimental group #2 included children scheduled for tonsillectomies, who had not been previously hospitalized, who participated in the play therapy and orientation program, and whose parents participated in the Pediatric Patient Parent Education Program. Two control groups composed of nonhospitalized children were also studied. All four groups were tested initially on the Children's Manifest Anxiety Scale (CMAS) seven days prior to hospital admission, again the evening of admission, and again seven days following discharge from the hospital. The Pediatric Patient Parent Education Program was an orientation program for parents, provided by hospital personnel, no later than seven days prior to admission to the hospital. The hospital treatment for children included simulation of anxiety-producing stimuli in a play situation, and actual visits to anxiety-producing settings in the hospital, including the x-ray room, recovery room, and surgery. When the data gathered from the CMAS was subjected to appropriate statistical analysis, no significant differences were found. The subjective reaction to the parent program and the experiences provided the children seemed to be positive. However, the techniques used did not produce significant changes in the levels of anxiety. It was recommended that changes be made in the anxiety measures and the patient population in further studies, to explore alternatives for dealing with the problem.

115. Conway, A. Oedipal concerns of a five-year-old girl during hospitalization. Maternal-Child Nursing Journal, 1973, 2(1), 39-48.

This article discusses the case of a five-year-old girl's oedipal reactions to her hospital stay for a diagnostic check-up. Her history, her relationship with her parents, and her regressive behaviors during hospitalization are described.

116. Conway, A. Oedipal concerns of hospitalized preschool girls. Maternal-Child Nursing Journal, 1975, 4(2), 75-82.

The author discusses the fears and apprehensions exhibited by children during the oedipal period of psychosexual development (e.g., fear of harm to the genitals, mutilation, and loss of parents' love) and maintains that such inner fears and conflicts are compounded by hospitalization. Specific examples are presented of the problems of preschool girls who were hospitalized during this stage of their development. It is pointed out that the nurse who is knowledgeable concerning this stage of development is in a position to recognize various manifestations of the Oedipus complex when they occur and provide appropriate intervention when needed. She can present reality to the child so that misconceptions can be avoided or corrected and can also help the parents understand their child's behavior and needs.

117. Conway, B. The effect of hospitalization on adolescence. Adolescence, 1971, 6, 77-92.

Many adolescents have problems in achieving independence, in maintaining control, and in coping with the unknown in the hospital setting. However, the type and extent of each adolescent's reaction is related to his individual adjustment to his environment. Thus, the nurse may assist the adolescent in having a more positive hospital experience by becoming acquainted with his personality traits, his emotional status, his social patterns, and his medical problems. It is suggested that the nurse apply his or her knowledge about care, as it pertains to the adolescent, in planning his care so that he maintains the maximum amount of control, and develops the most constructive attitude possible about his condition.

118. Cook, P. S. The admission of mothers to hospital with their young children. Medical Journal of Australia, 1970, 2(14), 650-651.

This article argues that the psychological and emotional damage caused in one year through lack of application of available knowledge about the care of children in hospital greatly exceeds that which all available child psychiatrists can undo in several years. There are many aspects of this problem, but some aspects of the application of this knowledge concern the design and administration of hospital buildings. The lack of sufficient nurses to provide adequate, let alone optimal, nursing care is a related consideration. In reviewing these problems the following recommendations are made: (1) In the planning of new hospitals and also in existing hospitals, provision should be made for the routine admission of mothers with their infants and young children, whenever possible; (2) Facilities for the above should include: (a) Mother-and-Child Rooms in which a mother can help to care for her infant or young child in the hospital ward; and (b) Care-by-Parent Units especially designed so that a mother can, in suitable cases, care for her sick child, with or without her other young children, whilst having the benefit of the hospital facilities for her sick child; and (3) This policy should be officially encouraged. Steps should be taken to study and overcome any obstacles to its implementation.

119. Cormier, P. N. Identification of typologies derived from child behaviors in the hospital as predictors of psychological upset (Doctoral dissertation, University of Virginia, 1975). Dissertation Abstracts International, 1976, 36(9-B), 4376.

The present study was designed to identify typologies from patterns of behavior of children in the hospital. It aimed to identify interpersonal typologies, focusing on the child rather than his measurable attributes as the entity which determines psychological upset. Thirty-two subjects, ages four through fifteen years, were observed in a hospital setting utilizing a time sampling method, recording behaviors on a forty-five item checklist, measuring thirty-two frequency variables and thirty-two global ratings. Results indicated that there were three patterns of behavior, divided into three factors which correlated specifically with the three stages of hospitalism: protest, despair and denial. Factor I typified Stage III--Denial; Factor II typified Stage II --Despair; and Factor III typified Stage I--Protest. Children in Factor I, Stage III were characterized by friendly, cooperative behavior, smiling, playing, but in limited contact with family members. Children in Factor II, Stage II were withdrawn and passive, exhibiting limited verbalization and frequent autoerotic behavior. Factor III, Stage I presented children who were irritable, complaining and aggressive, prone to extensive periods of crying and whimpering. Degree of psychological upset due to hospitalization did not demonstrate any significant difference with respect to age, sex, type and degree of illness, socioeconomic level, prior hospitalization and only slightly related to parental visiting situation.

120. Couture, C. J. The psychological response of young children to brief hospitalization and surgery: The role of parent-child contact and age (Doctoral dissertation, Boston University Graduate School, 1976). <u>Dissertation Abstracts International</u>, 1976, <u>37</u>(3-B), 1427.

The primary purpose of this study was to examine the role of varying degrees of parent-child contact and the child's age in determining the behavioral responses of young children to brief hospitalization for routine surgery. Thirty-one children, ranging in age from three years, one month to five years, eleven months, were studied under conditions of limited visiting, unlimited visiting and rooming-in by their parents. Behavioral observations of all children on a time sampling basis were made throughout the period of their hospitalization. The children were also rated, according to information provided by parents, on a behavior adjustment scale at the time of admission to hospital and again at one week and one month after discharge. Children under the pooled visiting conditions exhibited far more precipitous behavioral regression between the time of hospital admission and one week following discharge than did children under the parent rooming-in condition. In addition, while the "behavioral recovery rate" is approximately the same for these groups between one week and one month after discharge, the pooled visiting groups still had not returned at one month after discharge to their level of adjustment at the time of admission. The rooming-in group on the other hand had reached a level of developmental progression at one month after discharge relative to their behavioral adjustment level at admission.

121. Crawford, C. F., & Palm, M. L. Can I take my teddy bear? American Journal of Nursing, 1973, 73(2), 286-287.

This article describes a special hospital preparation program developed by the Evanston Hospital School of Nursing in which students visit families at home before scheduled admissions to pediatrics. Before a student calls the family to explain the program and arrange to visit, she gathers such factual data as the child's age, previous admissions, and reason for the present admission. The students take such visual aids as are appropriate and they vary their approach according to the child's age. She not only orients him on admission to the unit, but sees him throughout his hospitalization. She accompanies surgical patients to the operating room and takes care of them in the recovery room. She then writes a nursing care plan for each child to aid the rest of the nursing team. She telephones the family a few days after the child is discharged to see if hospitalization has changed the child's behavior. On the whole, the program has been enthusiastically accepted, as shown by the parents' replies to posthospital questionnaires.

122. Crocker, E. A review of the literature concerning the effects of hospitalization and illness on children or we know less than we think we do! Journal of the Association for the Care of Children in Hospitals, 1974, 3(2), 3-9.

The purpose of this paper is to outline the nature and results of the research that has focused on trying to determine the effects of hospitalization and illness on children. A major review of the literature in this field written by Vernon, Foley, Sipowicz and Schulman (1965) serves as the foundation for this article. A summary of their main findings as well as their evaluation of the calibre of the reseach is presented in Part I; in Part II, critical reviews of the major research reported in the literature since 1965 is presented.

123. Crocker, E. Play programs in pediatric settings. In E. Gellert (Ed.), Psychosocial aspects of pediatric care. New York: Grune & Stratton, 1978, 95-110.

Play is a universal phenomenon. All vertebrates, including humans, engage in play and game behavior that involves exploration of and interaction with things, people, and the environment. These behaviors, prevalent in all cultures, stimulate and foster cognitive, social, emotional, and physical development. The purpose of this chapter is to try to explain what play is, what things interfere with play, and what happens when humans cannot play. Such a discussion takes place within the framework of the importance of play programs for children in hospital, and provides a background for a rationale for such programs. The implications for play programs in various pediatric settings are discussed.

124. Crocker, E. Preparation for elective surgery: Does it make a difference. Journal of the Association for the Care of Children in Hospitals, 1980, 9(1), 3-11.

This study investigated the questions of whether preparation for surgery is beneficial and what type of preparation makes a difference. The unit selected for this project was a 27-bed, Ear, Eye, Nose and Throat unit housing children between four to 11 years old hospitalized for elective surgery. This study recorded two types of results--"objective" (physiological and behavioral) and "anecdotal," e.g., comments of preparation specialists and nursing staff. The study predicted that preparation would decrease children's anxiety. The fact that the prepared children showed less of a change in blood pressure supported this hypothesis, but the higher rate of vomiting in the same group went against the hypothesis. No other scientific data supported the general hypothesis, but the anecdotal comments of staff did refer to decreased anxiety and increased cooperation among children in the experimental group. It was predicted that younger children would be more anxious than older children and, in fact, this prediction was borne out, in the objective data, within the experimental group in terms of post-hospital measures. The hypothesis that the presence of parents would have a positive effect on the reduction of anxiety in their children was not supported by any of the objective data. The comments of nursing staff, however, did indicate that children whose parents were present appeared to be less anxious. Also, by looking at and comparing children who had never been in the hospital before with children who had experienced one or more hospitalizations, there was some evidence that children in the control group who could be viewed as "experienced," in fact, showed more signs of anxiety than "novices."

125. Crocker, E. Reactions of children in health care encounters: Programs that can make a difference. In G. C. Robinson and H. F. Clarke (Eds.), The hospital care of children: A review of contemporary issues. Oxford: Oxford University Press, 1980, 90-107.

Almost every situation that affects adults and children has within it the potential for growth. Health care encounters are no different; they need not be traumatic but instead can be constructive experiences. In every instance, the overall aim of health care settings and personnel should be to try to ensure that children and families do not lose out either physiologically or psychosocially--that they gain in terms of continued growth and development and the pursuit of normal activities, increased understanding of why they were there and what happened, and new knowledge about what to do in the future (for illness, to prevent or treat accidents, and to promote health). The "pediatric paradox" has been that we have known what types of programs and policies can make positive differences in people's abilities to cope with illness or surgery but we have not begun to practice what we know. Implementation of programs for parental involvement, preparation, therapeutic play and school can help bridge the gap between what we know and what we do and can lead to positive feelings about health care encounters.

126. Dadich, K. S. An eleven year old girl's use of control while immobilized in halo-femoral traction. Maternal-Child Nursing Journal, 1972, 1(1), 67-74.

This article describes the case of an eleven year old girl immobilized for correction of scoliosis. The child's coping mechanisms used to deal with the anxiety resulting from immobilization and hospitalization were directed toward attaining self-control and control of other persons. Self-control was achieved through a variety of methods: (1) denial; (2) cognitive mastery; (3) withdrawal; (4) compulsivity; and (5) verbalizations of fears and fantasies. Control of other persons was expressed through the use of verbal commands. These two areas are discussed separately.

127. Danilowicz, D. A., & Gabriel, H. P. Postoperative reactions in children: "Normal" and abnormal responses after cardiac surgery. American Journal of Psychiatry, 1971, 128, 185-188.

The authors note the acute responses of 68 children who underwent cardiac operations and describe in detail the grossly abnormal reactions of four, discussing the possible predisposing factors in three of the four children. The major normal reactions were divided into four groups: anxiety, anger, cooperation, and compliance. The relation of these reactions to preoperative personality and preparation and to postoperative medical complications remains uncertain. Careful evaluations of personality, before and after children undergo major operations, are needed to produce information that will be useful in preparing other children for similar operations.

128. Dart, R. J. Reducing stress in young children: Effects of mother's picture and voice recordings on response to hospitalization (Doctoral dissertation, University of Waterloo, 1980). Dissertation Abstracts International, 1980, 41(3-B), 1104-1105.

An interventive program was developed to provide the separated child with a kind of "automated surrogate mother"--a photograph and a voice-recording of the individual child's mother, presented via a toy television set. Sixteen three- and four-year-old tonsillectomy-adenoidectomy patients were randomly assigned to each of three experiemental groups, blocking by age. All 48 subjects had constant access to the experiemental toy television set throughout the 48-hour hospitalization. However, each experimental group was presented with different material via the toy television: Mother Group subjects were presented with mother's photograph and mother's voice-recording of the child's favorite stories, rhymes and songs, Stranger Group subjects with an unfamiliar "storylady's" photograph and the storylady's voice-recording of the child's favorite stories, rhymes and songs, and Control Group subjects with a landscape photograph and an audio-recording of a collection of classical music. As predicted, results indicated that, relative to Stranger and Control Group subjects, Mother Group subjects showed more positive reactions to hospitalization. Also, compared with Stranger and Control Group treatments, the Mother Group treatment resulted in higher frequencies of play, curiosity-attention and positive affect and lower frequencies of dependency, aggression, withdrawal, self-orientation, and negative affect. Following hospital discharge, Mother Group subjects showed significantly less disturbed regressive behavior than subjects in the other experimental groups.

129. Davenport, H. T., & Werry, J. S. The effect of general anesthesia, surgery and hospitalization upon the behavior of children. American Journal of Orthopsychiatry, 1970, 40(5), 806-824.

This study compared the behavior of 145 United States and Canadian one to fifteen year olds undergoing tonsillectomy to that of sibs or normal controls. Behavioral data was obtained by a questionnaire administered to mothers of subjects before surgery and two weeks later. Contrary to the findings of several recent studies, no significant evidence of post-hospitalization upset was found, nor were differences discovered between the Canadian and the United States groups.

130. David, N. Play: A nursing diagnostic tool. Maternal-Child Nursing Journal, 1973, 2(1), 49-56.

This paper describes the patterns of play exhibited by a six-year-old boy during his hospitalization. Greg was admitted to a metropolitan children's hospital for treatment of burns, classified as second and third degree and covering approximately ten per cent of his body. His previous medical history was negative, and this was his first hospitalization. Greg's play was the best means for the nurse to understand what he was experiencing and how he perceived various situations.

Furthermore, play was used by Greg as his best coping device throughout his hospitalization. Play was the part of his life that he could modify if he wished.

131. Davis, J. L. Preoperative program prepares children for surgery. AORN Journal, 1977, 26(2), 249-256.

Preoperative preparation for the pediatric patient and family is the first step toward demonstrating the warm, loving, and caring environment of the hospital. If preparation is begun after hospital admission, the child and family may not have dealt with preconceived fears and fantasies. Also, the child may have already experienced painful procedures for which he was unprepared. This article describes an effective preoperative information program initiated at Hope Haven Children's Hospital, Jacksonville, Florida, in 1976. Several goals were established: (1) to acquaint interested adults and children with the usual sequence of events encountered with a surgical experience; (2) to provide information to assist persons in coping with a potential emotionally traumatizing situation; (3) to communicate a sincere interest in accomplishing individualized nursing care throughout an anticipated hospitalization or a hospitalization that is in progress; and (4) to acquaint parents and families with policies and procedures of this hospital. The program is described and discussed.

132. Deakers, L. P. Continuity of family-centered nursing care between the hospital and the home. Nursing Clinics of North America, 1972, 7(1), 83-93.

Comprehensive, family-centered care is a global approach to pediatric nursing and must consider the total experience of illness--both in the hospital and in the community. The professional nurse must recognize her responsibility to the family and the community and insure that continuity of care is provided. The degree of continuity provided depends upon the ability of the health team to work together. The professional nurse must identify the family's learning needs and with their participation prepare a written discharge plan. Teaching is an integral part of the nurse's role in discharge planning. Instruction sessions should be appropriately planned for the family. Before discharge the health team must determine if follow-up care by a community agency is necessary. Hospital and community agency administrations must recognize the need for staff development in the areas of discharge planning and follow-up care or continuity of care will not prevail.

133. Dearden, R. The psychiatric aspects of the case study sample. In M. Stacey (Ed.), Hospitals, children and their families: The report of a pilot study. London: Routledge & Kegan Paul, Ltd., 1970, 55-84.

The evidence presented in this chapter relates to a sample of children who entered one of two hospitals for tonsillectomy and adenoidectomy. Almost all of the children in the study exhibited a deterioration in behavior as reported by their mothers immediately upon discharge. Nineteen of the thirty-six had recovered a satisfactory pre-hospital position six months later. Ten had not, and were termed disturbed. Seven were isolated as maladjusted, showing high reported behavior disturbance before going to hospital and remaining in a high category throughout the seven months of the survey. A number of factors which seemed likely to provide a measure of vulnerability to hospitalization are examined.

134. Deasy, P. F. The special needs of children in hospital. Journal of the Irish Medical Association, 1978, 71(16), 521-522.

This article outlines policies and services as they apply to hospitalized children in Ireland. Several recent hospital surveys and policy reports are reviewed. The author concludes with recommendations and suggestions for areas needing continued research.

135. Demaio, D. J. Body image concerns of a six year old boy. Maternal-Child Nursing Journal, 1978, 7(3), 175-184.

This article presents the case study of a six year old boy, Brian, hospitalized for bone fracture following an auto accident. The author discusses this child's concerns about his body image. They were most frequently related to the anatomical structure of his body and less frequently related to self-representational concerns. The expression of self-feeling concerns was concurrent with expressions of body representation concerns. Brian's developmental level was a major factor that accounted for the expression of numerous body image concerns while hospitalized. The body image is emphasized during latency especially when the child is ill since illness draws attention to the body. Brian's hospitalization included immobilization, imposed dependency, separation from home and family, and placement in a strange, threatening, and often painful environment. The reasons for these factors were poorly understood by Brian. He undoubtedly viewed the hospitalization as punishment for being bad. Brian's ability to verbalize his fears enabled him to recognize alterations in his body and in his sense of self. He attempted to reduce his anxiety by repeating frightening situaions in play until he mastered them and by verbalization of fantasies and fears in order to cope with them.

136. Dicker, K. Six days to sunday. Nursing Times, 1973, 69(9), 309.

The author presents her personal views of how pediatric wards have changed in the past 40 years. She makes comparisons between her current experience as a sick child's nurse to those experiences she encountered during her own hospitalization at age eight.

137. Digby, M. The hospital play therapist. Child: Care, Health and Development, 1975, 1(4), 233-237.

This article discusses the role and responsibilities of a hospital play therapist. The author notes the following responsibilities of these individuals: (1) Provision of play and activities on the ward and in the playroom; (2) Selection and care of play equipment; (3) Forming a helpful relationship with parents and supplementing the mother's care; (4) She may request that the family be referred to the social worker; and (5) She supports medical treatment and the medical-nursing staff. As a hospital play therapist associated with the Save the Children Fund, the author discusses some of her personal experiences with play therapy.

138. Dittemore, I. Play utilized by a burned child. Maternal-Child Nursing Journal, 1973, 2(3), 203-214.

This article presents a transcript of a play session with a six-year-old girl who had suffered severe burns at the age of four. This play session took place in the early postoperative period during the child's fourth hospitalization in a five-bed ward on the pediatric unit of a large hospital. Two other children were present in the ward at the time.

139. Doak, S., & Wallace, N. The doctors wear pajamas. Journal of the Association for the Care of Children in Hospitals, 1975, 3(3), 8-13, 20.

The Child Life Program of Yale-New Haven Hospital provides activity and education programs to meet the developmental needs of hospitalized children. The child life staff, trained in group skills, child development and education direct daily group play and activity programs for specific age groups, i.e., the toddler-preschool, school age and adolescent patients, in large playrooms located on the division. Hospital play provides an important tool for children to use in coping with hospitalization. Through group hospital play, children gain support from their peers. The group sanctions expressions of anger, frustration, and fear, and hospital play techniques provide acceptable channels for these feelings. Follow-up through further play, direct clarification and communication with medical staff caring for the patient, helps to insure that problems and feelings revealed in the sessions are acknowledged and handled. Hospital play is a vital component of total pediatric care. It is a unique and essential form of play which should be provided periodically throughout the child's hospital stay, and which parents may find helpful to continue at home.

140. Douglas, J. W. B. Early hospital admissions and later disturbances of behaviour and learning. Developmental Medicine and Child Neurology, 1975, 17(4), 456-480.

This study provides strong and unexpected evidence that one admission to hospital of more than a week's duration or repeated admissions before the age of five years (in particular between six months and four years) are associated with an increased risk of behaviour disturbance and poor reading in adolescence. The children who have experienced these early admissions are more troublesome out of class, more likely to be delinquent and more likely to show unstable job-patterns than those who are not admitted in the first five years. They include a high proportion of poor readers, though this is partly explained by poor application to work in the classroom. In contrast, nervous, shy or withdrawn behaviour is not more frequently reported in adolescence among children who have had early hospital-admissions.

141. Dowd, E. L., Novak, J. C., & Ray, E. J. Releasing the hospitalized child from restraints. MCN: American Journal of Maternal Child Nursing, 1977, 2(6), 370-373.

This article reports on the observations and interactions of the authors with 20 hospitalized children requiring restraint. The needs for and responses to restraint varied among the children studied, but some definite patterns were noted. All of the children under 18 months cried and whined but displayed less struggling. When infants were temporarily freed of their encumbrances for the first time, they initially remained immobile. As they experienced being set free more often, however, their activity levels progressively increased as did their protest behaviors when their restraints were restored. In contrast, the degree of protest in the toddlers and preschoolers decreased with each episode of removing and restoring restraints. A program of verbal and nonverbal techniques was found to be effective in helping restrained pediatric patients. The staff removed the child's restraints for at least ten minutes every two hours. The restraints were then restored as loosely as possible, changing the child's position. Throughout both phases of the intervention the staff talked soothingly to the child and offered him explanations. The staff also used a doll with restraints for explaining to both toddlers and preschoolers the reason for their own limitations.

142. Downey, T. J. All my times in the hospital: A child remembers. American Journal of Nursing, 1974, 74(12), 2196-2198.

This article describes a little boy's story of his hospital experiences told to, and written by his mother.

143. Drexler, C. A four-year-old boy experiences surgery for a genital defect. Maternal-Child Nursing Journal, 1975, 4(3), 197-205.

The author describes the experiences of a four-year-old Black male who underwent surgery to repair a genital defect. The article focuses on his preparation for hospitalization and surgery and the major sources of anxiety he encountered. The behaviors he demonstrated in his efforts to deal with his experiences are also discussed.

144. Droske, S. C. Children's behavioral changes following hospitalization--have we prepared the patient? Journal of the Association for the Care of Children in Hospitals, 1978, 7(2), 3-7.

This article discusses the three stages of separation anxiety (i.e., protest, despair, and denial) observed in hospitalized children, and describes how these may be reflected in their posthospitalization behaviors. Frequent posthospitalization behavior changes observed in children include: (a) increased demands upon parents for attention; (b) increased intensity of reaction to temporary separations; and (c) sleep disorders. Research showing that parents react with anxiety to such behavior changes in their children is reviewed, and ways in which hospital staff may help parents deal with their children's posthospitalization adjustment are discussed.

145. Duffy, J. C. Emotional reactions of children to hospitalization. Minnesota Medicine, 1972, 55(12), 1168-1170.

In recent years the child who enters the hospital can be certain of a thorough clinical investigation, whatever his presenting problem, but may find his emotional needs unmet. Even our outstanding scientific pediatric services can place a child in a situation which is excessively impersonal, concerned too little with his feelings. Children may have emotional reactions to hospitalization during their stay and/or manifest these reactions after they have left the hospital. The literature on a child's emotional response to hospitalization had, for the most part, explored various explanations for these responses. In this article, the author explores the following issues: unfamiliarity, separation, sensory-motor restriction, the child's concept of the hospital, age, family, parents, and other related issues.

146. Duran, M. T. Family-centered care and the adolescent's quest for self-identity. Nursing Clinics of North America, 1972, 7(1), 65-73.

Adolescence is a definite period of development and has identifiable needs, resources, and goals. The nurse, in order to be a therapeutic agent, must be capable of identifying them in her patients and utilizing her intervention skills to promote independence in the adolescent. The parent is a resource for her intervention, and often an active, contributing agent in the maintenance and growth of his child's self-identity through a period of adjustment. Illness provokes many varying emotional responses from individuals. It can be a growth experience for the adolescent, if his continuance for independence and self-identity is not stifled but supported by providing family-centered nursing care.

147. Dzik, M. A. The use of motility by a preschool boy during hospitalization. Maternal-Child Nursing Journal, 1974, 3(3), 169-179.

This paper is concerned with the use of motility by Jimmy, a five year old child, during his fourth hospitalization for repair of a cleft lip. Motility was an important factor in Jimmy's adjustment to the hospital experience. In the initial period, he seemed to move for the sake of movement. This activity corresponded to the movement described in the literature as that related to the id and representing a means of tension discharge. Evidence of ego involvement was also observed. Jimmy was able to hold his impulses under control. Although he wanted to leave the hospital on the first postoperative morning, he contented himself with gazing out the door. Throughout the hospitalization, at the time of the lip care procedure he lay very still and followed directions about position regardless of his discomfort. Jimmy's physical actions seemed to be more than simply movement: they seemed to be the physical counterpart of his mental state. His physical actions also served as stimulators for change: when Jimmy cried, he not only relieved his tension, but he also caused a change in his environment. Through the motor acts of play, he worked on his feelings about separation and powerlessness. Thus, motor behavior served as a therapeutic tool.

148. Earthrowl, B., & Stacey, M. Social class and children in hospital. Social Science and Medicine, 1977, 11(2), 83-88.

It is sometimes proposed that working class parents do not understand the social and emotional needs of their children in hospital. A survey of over 1000 children discharged from Welsh hospitals in 1972 does not uphold such propositions. The only major differences to emerge among the classes were associated with economic differences. Members of lower occupational groups less often have cars, have greater difficulty both in obtaining and in paying for transport, and are more likely to suffer a loss of income if the household head absents himself from work to ease the home situation or to be with the child in hospital. Some class differences emerged in the routes whereby children reached hospital and there were some hints that higher economic classes used the hospital services differently from others. But there were few class differences found about what were felt by parents to be the needs of children in hospital. Little variation by social class was found in the views of parents about the importance of explaining hospital to children, or in their wishes for information about their children, or in the harm possibly caused by lack of regular visiting, or in their efforts to maintain regular contact. Middle class parents were more able to obtain information which satisfied them about their children and working class parents were less likely to ask for information. On the whole, members of all classes wanted the same goals for their children, but were differentially able, partly for cultural, but largely for economic reasons, to achieve these goals.

149. Eckhardt, L. O., & Prugh, D. G. Preparing children psychologically for painful medical and surgical procedures. In E. Gilbert (Ed.), Psychosocial aspects of pediatric care. New York: Grune & Stratton, 1978, 75-82.

The psychological preparation of children for the stress related to painful medical and surgical procedures is a complicated task. This challenge is compounded by the ever-changing cognitive and emotional responses that spring from the child's level of physical, cognitive, psychosexual, and psychosocial development. The child's genetic endowment, his developmental capacities, the degree of supportiveness offered by his family environment, his past experiences, and his psychological defenses will play major roles in determining the nature of the outcome of his reaction to stressful stimuli. The role of the physician and other health professionals involved in the care of the child in hospital is discussed.

150. Edison, C. C. Reintegration of ego functioning during recovery from a cerebral insult. Maternal-Child Nursing Journal, 1978, 7(2), 87-98.

The early period of adolescence is a period of vulnerability. When illness and hospitalization are added to the sphere of the early adolescent's experience, it becomes necessary for him to assume additional stresses which hold high emotional significance. This article presents the case study of a twelve and a half year old boy whose psychological adaptation in the recovery process that followed a cerebral vascular accident is evaluated in terms of the phenomena of sudden, traumatic enforced regression. Identification of a definitive pattern of behavior revealed the boy's initial primitive, infantile ego responses and successive evidence of progress in the reintegration of ego function.

151. Eikeland, T. A case of conditioned fear in a two-year-old boy after tonsillectomy. Acta Otolarynogologica, 1973, 76(5), 377-380.

Some behavioural sequelae after tonsillectomy in a two-year-old boy are described. It is made an essential point that the pre-verbal or pre-logical child (0-5 years) is especially vulnerable to hospital practices. The behavioural sequelae observed in this patient are interpreted and treated according to learning theory in contrast to the global psychoanalytical ways of treating such phenomena. Some sort of conditioned phobic reactions are supposed to occur in most pre-verbal children during hospitalization and parents should be informed to observe the behaviour of their children after they have been discharged from hospital.

152. Elmassian, B. J. A practical approach to communicating with children through play. MCN: American Journal of Maternal Child Nursing Journal, 1979, 4(4), 238-240.

Getting through to a child in the face of a frightening situation is first and foremost therapeutic for the child. A secondary benefit is that it can help direct the child's self-expression into less disruptive, more acceptable channels. This article details how play situations can be used to help children facing frightening situations. Several case study examples are presented along with suggestions for handling conflicts with children.

153. Epstein, M. H., & Harris, J., Jr. Children with chronic pain: Can they be helped? Pediatric Nursing, 1978, 4(1), 42-44.

Chronic pain in children is treatable and should not be ignored. A child may express his discomfort by irritability, behavior disorders, and ultimately impaired school performance. It is important to prevent the pain from causing permanent damage to the child's physical and emotional development. The use of a comprehensive treatment center concept utilizing the latest medical methods of pain control, coupled with a team approach to physical and emotional rehabilitation appears to be a promising approach to a complex problem.

154. Erickson, F. Stress in the pediatric ward. Maternal-Child Nursing Journal, 1972, 1(2), 113-116.

The author discusses a hospitalized child's preoccupation with violence and death. The child's anxieties included fear of suffocation, what happens to other child patients, the medical rounds of a doctor, and fear of mutilation or disfigurement. An understanding of these anxieties is considered basic for those who work with children in hospitals.

155. Eyres, P. J. The role of the nurse in family-centered nursing care. Nursing Clinics of North America, 1972, 7(1), 27-39.

The major concern within this article is that nurses must have a personal commitment to their own life experiences and to a philosophy of nursing if they are to be nurses. The role of the nurse in family-centered care is viewed as a dynamic process arising out of a blending of appropriate cues inspired by the interaction of uniquely individual personalities. Climate and therapeutic use of the self have been much discussed in relation to the nurse's role. The concept of ombudsman represents a more innovative component, and one that deserves more attention from nurses. The melding of these components and the admonition to nurses to be yourself and become involved will represent for many a new dimension in the role of the nurse providing family-centered care.

156. Fagin, C. M., & Nusbaum, J. G. Parental visiting privileges in pediatric units: A survey. Journal of Nursing Administration, 1978, 8(3), 24-27.

Questionnaries were sent to 1,154 hospitals throughout the United States to identify the extent to which unlimited visiting for parents is permitted on pediatric services. Of these, 636 returned responses that were usable for data tabulations. Sixty-two percent of the sample indicated that parents were permitted twenty-four-hour visiting in pediatric units. In relation to unit size, census, age of children, diagnosis, or length of stay, no differences were found between hospitals that do and those that do not permit twenty-four-hour parental visiting. However, there were interesting regional variations in the percentage of hospitals permitting twenty-four-hour visiting. The lowest percentage of hospitals permitting twenty-four-hour visiting on pediatric units was found in the Northeast Region. This region has the greatest percentage of highly educated physicians and nurses and the oldest traditions in both fields.

157. Fassler, D. Experiences with children and books in hospital settings. Journal of the Association for the Care of Children in Hospitals, 1977, 6(1), 12-16.

One of the best ways to help a child cope with the threatening experience of hospitalization is by providing an outlet for feelings, emotions, and thoughts. In this way, a caring adult can better deal with the child's actual concerns. Children's books can be a valuable tool in aiding this process of communication. Books from different genres offer children the opportunity to project fears on to story characters and discuss feelings openly. In the course of work on several pediatric wards, this author has found a number of books particularly useful for this purpose. This paper discusses several of the publications most valuable in reaching hospitalized children.

158. Ferguson, F., & Robertson, J. Making hospital preparation child-centered (with a little help from Emily). Journal of the Association for the Care of Children in Hospitals, 1979, 8(2), 27-31.

At Alberta Children's Hospital, several innovative ideas for the preparation of children to hospitals have been implemented as described in this article. Drawing on the coordinated efforts of the Recreation/Child Life Department and the Nursing Department, the process consists of several phases, commencing prior to admission and carrying right through until discharge. The "thread" that draws all the parts together is a whimsical character named Emily. A coloring book developed around this character has become an important part of the Nursing Department's Preadmission Visiting Program. At the time of a preadmission home visit several days prior to the child's arrival at the hospital, a nurse gives a copy of the coloring book to the child and explains each picture as it depicts Emily's experience at the hospital. During hospitalization the child again meets Emily in the form of a puppet show and through play acting. Following surgery the child is given a badge emblazoned with Emily's picture. The efforts of the staff to use this character to reduce traumatic hospital experiences among children has met with success as reported by children and their parents.

159. Fines, B. The native child in hospital. Dimensions in Health Service, 1979, 56(5), 62-64.

This article discusses the special problems of native children admitted to the Health Sciences Centre in Winnipeg. The difficulties encountered in using interpreters is discussed, including issues of confidentiality. The frequency of various diseases commonly encountered are outlined along with some discussion of their probable origins. The author also provides information on some of the special techniques used to reduce the stress of hospitalization among native children including diet changes to include familiar foods, a game room, and the use of child life therapists.

160. Foust, L. A. The concerns of a ten year old boy threatened with body image disruption due to a reconstructive craniofacial surgery. Maternal-Child Nursing Journal, 1980, 9(1), 37-48.

The purpose of this case study was to determine what influence the threat of body image disruption had on the behavior of one ten-year-old boy (David), hospitalized for major reconstructive craniofacial surgery. In the preoperative period David's major concerns were related to loss of mental function as an outcome of surgery, and about receiving injections. Playing with needle and syringe in conjunction with his teddy bear in the preoperative period noticeably decreased his anxieties about injections. Postoperatively Davids's concerns focused on the injured part. Initially in the postoperative period David's reactions to changed body image and to the intensive care environment were global and regressive in nature. Gradually, as he touched, explored and moved his body parts, re-organization of disrupted body image was initiated. David gradually began to change the focus of his attention from concerns related to mutilation to concerns about appearance. By the day of discharge appearance was David's total concern.

161. Frank, J. L. A weekly group meeting for children on a pediatric ward: Therapeutic and pracitcal functions. International Journal of Psychiatry in Medicine, 1977-78, 8(3), 267-283.

This article describes the functions of a weekly group meeting for school aged hospitalized children led by a child psychiatrist. Over a one year period, the 40-bed pediatric ward in an urban hospital had over 1,000 admissions, the average length of stay was 10 days. About 50% of the children came from nearby Black and Puerto Rican ghetto areas. Knowledge gained from the children was used for therapeutic purposes within the group and for teaching the inpatient pediatric staff how hospitalized children's behavior reflects their inner thoughts and feelings. Aspects of the children's behavior and verbal productions in the group are discussed from a psychodynamic viewpoint. Conflict, ambivalence, fantasy distortion, denial, and displacement are exemplified as is the children's ever-present need to simultaneously express, defend against, and master anxiety. Questions are raised about outcome and future avenues of investigation.

162. Freeman, A. A day in the life of a child in hospital. Nursing Times, 1976, 72(50), 1974-1976.

In order to see what could be learned from devoting a day to carrying out the nursing care of one child, a nurse arranged to have a day without any other responsibilities on the ward. A nurse's work is often job-oriented instead of patient-oriented, and this experiment was designed to help nursing staff become more sensitive to young patients' needs. The venture proved rewarding in that a relationship seemed to be formed between the nurse, the baby and her mother that was of benefit to all.

163. Frieberg, K. H. How parents react when their child is hospitalized. American Journal of Nursing, 1972, 72(7), 1270-1272.

This report details the responses of 25 mothers asked to discuss the hospitalization experience of their children and the effects it had had on the child and family in the first few days after discharge. The 25 children, 16 boys and 9 girls, ranged in age from 15 months to nine years. Statistics on race and social status were also obtained. Subjects, however, were chosen simply by the mother's willingness to comply with an interview rather than by these other criteria. Results showed that: (1) the mothers perceived that their children were unhappy and frightened while in the hospital; (2) the mothers reported that all children had shown various degrees of crying, screaming, or belligerent behavior toward hospital personnel and procedures; (3) after hospitalization many of the children in the study group had difficulties recuperating from the traumatic experience of hospitalization itself as well as from their illness; (4) parental reactions to the hospitalization were also laced with fear and anxiety: all mothers said that they had felt some degree of uneasiness, fear, or anxiety while their child was hospitalized, even if a specific frightening incident had not occurred; (5) fifteen mothers had misunderstood or lacked knowledge about diagnosis, treatment, and follow-up; and (6) when one child in a family was hospitalized, the family life was considerably disrupted, according to the 25 mothers interviewed.

164. Fujita, M. T. The impact of illness or surgery on the body image of the child. Nursing Clinics of North America, 1972, 7(4), 641-649.

A great deal of interest has been generated in the past twenty years regarding hospitalization and the child. Studies on the emotional aspects of certain surgeries and the effects of disease on childhood adjustment have brought about significant change in children's hospitals and hospital procedures such as liberalized visiting hours, rooming-in facilities, preoperative visits, more pleasant surroundings, and individualized nursing care. This article discusses the impact of illness on body image. The body image of the hospitalized child is influenced by the attitude of others around him, his stage of development, and the illness event. The quality of the child's relationship with significant others is crucial in reintegration of his body image. A case study is presented to illustrate the impact of acute hospitalization.

165. Galdston, R., & Hughes, M. C. Pediatric hospitalization as crisis intervention. American Journal of Psychiatry, 1972, 129(6), 721-725.

The presence of psychiatric illness among children who have been hospitalized for signs and symptoms of organic disease constitutes one of the more difficult therapeutic problems confronting the psychiatrist in general hospital practice. Hospitalization of a child precipitates a crisis in family life regardless of the cuase. The disruption of routine, the anxieties at separation, and the fantasies and fears of illness and its sequelae are some of the factors that actuely threaten both the child and his parents. The authors describe a follow-up clinic for pediatric patients who have been hospitalized; an attempt is made to transform the acute crisis of hospitalization into a therapeutic relationship aimed at ameliorating intrapsychic and intrafamily problems. This approach has been successful both with patients with demonstrable organic disease and those without such disease.

166. Galligan, A. C. Books for the hospitalized child. American Journal of Nursing, 1975, 75(12), 2164-2166.

Books can have a positive effect on a child's mental health, development, and perception of life. This article lists books for children the author feels can provide the following benefits: (1) comfort and security; (2) quiet relaxation; (3) information and clarification; (4) self-awareness; (5) amelioration of withdrawal; and (6) imaginative thinking.

167. Garber, B., & Polsky, R. Follow-up study of hospitalized adolescents. Archives of General Psychiatry, 1970, 22, 179-187.

This article presents a preliminary report of a study initiated in 1968, to follow-up adolescents hospitalized at the Institute for Psychosomatic and Psychiatric Research and Training in Chicago from 1958 to 1968. The objectives of the study were: (1) To describe the adolescent population and its hospital courses; (2) To extract variables which may be correlated with the hospital course and functioning upon follow-up; (3) To determine what has happened to former adolescent patients and the status of their current functioning; and (4) To get some idea of their reaction to and their utilization of the hospital and the adolescent program. Preliminary data are presented, and the next step will be to develop scales for assessing with reliability the current functioning of the follow-up sample. Analysis of the hospital course in relation to the assessments of current functioning is planned.

168. Gardner, G. G., & Simkins, R. A. Does it really matter what nurses wear in the intensive care unit? MCN: American Journal of Maternal Child Nursing, 1976, 1(4), 239-242.

What a nurse wears and its effect on total patient care, especially when the patients are children, has in recent years become a prominent point of conjecture. Various studies on general pediatric wards and on pediatric surgical and clinical research units have found that children are often less anxious, while parents find the atmosphere more relaxed and nurses more approachable when nurses wear colorful outfits. Although this idea has been accepted in many hospitals for general pediatric wards, pediatric intensive care units (ICUs) have been another matter. This article discusses a study conducted to find out what attitudes toward nursing were. One of the major findings was that the clothes worn by nurses were not as important as many hospital staff commonly believe. Rather, excellence of nursing care and a friendly reassuring attitude are the important factors.

169. Gerbing, D. D. Putting play to work in pediatrics. MCN: American Journal of Maternal Child Nursing, 1977, 2(6), 387.

This author outlines his use of a crossword puzzle as a teaching tool and assessment guide for a 15-year-old boy with renal medulllary cystic disease. The puzzle which uses terms specific to the boy's hospitalization experience and illness helped the author to assess the boy's fine motor coordination and cognitive development as he filled in the answers. Words such as sick, hospital, and renal were very difficult for this 15-year-old. The final facets of this and similar play activities are that the patient has fun doing it, the activity provides an opportunity for one to give additional bedside care, and the patient feels comforted in knowing of another's genuine concern about him. No matter what the illness or condition, a similar individualized puzzle can do the same job--and perhaps even more.

170. Gerhart, S. M. A preschool child's use of language in coping with hospitalization. Maternal-Child Nursing Journal, 1979, 8(1), 39-47.

Andrea, the four year old subject of this paper, had been in good physical health prior to first admission to hospital and had experienced normal developmental milestones. Of significance was the fact that she had begun to articulate simple words at eight months of age. During a routine physical examination at ten months of age, a heart murmur was detected. Hospitalization followed. Andrea utilized expressions of language in her efforts to maintain self esteem while alternating between autonomy and dependency during two hospitalizations. This important feature of the subject's coping mechanisms is discussed and examples of how language was used during the traumatic experience of hospitalization reviewed.

171. Gibbons, M. B. When parents ask about play: Selecting toys and activities. Pediatric Nursing, 1977, 3(6), 19-22.

The adult has his vocation; in much the same way, play is the child's daily work. Play occupies most of the child's waking hours and is the way in which he learns about the world. Play is essential to the child, for it promotes his physical, intellectual, social and emotional development. This article describes types of play, and examines play patterns and play stages to serve as guidelines for nurses and parents as a key to understanding the appropriate materials to offer a child at each stage of growth and development.

172. Gildea, J. H., & Quirk, T. R. Assessing the pain experience in children. Nursing Clinics of North America, 1977, 12(4), 631-637.

Various biologic, sociologic, and psychologic definitions of pain exist in the literature today. Most relevant to nursing practice is this definition: "Pain is whatever the experiencing person says it is and exists whenever he says it does." Since infants and children are vulnerable to the pain experience, this definition is applicable for the pediatric nurse. The perception of pain and the expressive behaviors that are indicative of it are the result of the interaction of influential factors. Nursing intervention is possible only after a complete assessment of the pain experience is made. This paper discusses five factors to be considered when assessing the pain experience of infants and children: (1) Developmental level; (2) Parental attitudes; (3) Effects of hospitalization; (4) Symbolic meaning; (5) Physiologic response.

173. Glaser, H. H. The hospital as an environment for children and their families. Pediatric Annals, 1972, 1(3), 10-22.

This article discusses many of the environmental design considerations important to the optimal functioning of a children's hospital. Attention is focused on the following topics: (1) alternatives to hospitalization; (2) the relationship between the hospital and the community; (3) environments for children at different developmental levels; (4) the family's place in the hospital; (5) designing for staff satisfaction; and (6) application of of developmental principles to design of pediatric nursing units.

174. Gnus, M. A therapeutic play session in a health center. Maternal-Child Nursing Journal, 1973, 2(3), 197-201.

This article presents the case history of a five and one-half year old preschool child, Brad, hospitalized for an ear disorder. The author discusses the use of play therapy in helping Brad cope with his illness and its treatment in a hospital setting. Techniques for aiding hospitalized children in general through play therapy are discussed.

175. Gohsman, B., & Yunck, M. Dealing with the threats of hospitalization. Pediatric Nursing, 1979, 5(5), 32-35.

Hospitalization for surgery creates a series of real, imagined, or potential threats for the child and his parents. The type of threat can be classified in categories of physical harm or bodily injury, separation, the possibility of unpleasant surprise, uncertainty about the limits for behavior, and relative loss of control. Because of these threats, the child and his parents are under varying degrees of stress. Nurses can provide information, instruction and other support measures to minimize stress. This article discusses the following threatening situations as major causes of stress during hospitalization: admission, bedtime, receiving the pre-operative medication, leaving for the operating room, and returning from the recovery room.

176. Goldman, M., Sponseller, D., & Ream, B. A play program in a community hospital? MCN: American Journal of Maternal Child Nursing, 1978, 3(1), 42-45.

This article describes a play program developed at Pontiac General Hospital through a unqiue team approach in cooperation with Oakland University. The play program is composed of two main components: child play and parent education. The play component includes activities in a colorful playroom for children who are ambulatory and play at the bedside for those children who are unable to come to the room. Activities scheduled for the playroom are duplicated as much as possible in the individual rooms. The play component includes infant stimulation--auditory, visual, tactile, and motor. Parent eduation is achieved primarily through informal dialogue with the play staff when other staff members are working with the child or in the playroom itself when the parent accompanies the child. A parent education booklet is also distributed. Parents are provided with information concerning children's responses--both immediate and post-hospital--to hospitalization; normal growth and development; and the value of play. Case studies are presented to illustrate how this play program has been successfully implemented.

177. Goslin, E. R. Hospitalization as a life crisis for the preschool child: A critical review. Journal of Community Health, 1978, 3(4), 321-346.

This review of the literature on the psychological effects of hospitalization on children reveals that it has not increased substantially in quality or quantity over the past decade. Recent research supports the contentions that children between the ages of six months and four years are especially vulnerable to upset but are also more amenable to change and growth than other age groups. Maternal separation appears to be the primary stressor, but the presence of emotional disturbance prior to hospitalization and the child's level of cognitive development at the time may also be significant factors. Attempts to prepare children for hospitalization and surgery have met with some success, but not for preschool children. The need for some comprehensive theoretical perspective on which to base research is evident. Studies to date appear to have been based either on the concept of "anticipatory worry" or on some form of modeling theory. The author suggests that hospitalization can be considered as a life crisis for a child, a crisis that may result in blocks or distortions in his development if not mastered properly. Crisis theory provides a meaningful and useful model for understanding the experience of hospitalization for young children and for providing a basis for intervention. The psychopathology present in some children and their families is made apparent during such a crisis as hospitalization; this may present the only time when they are accessible to mental health professionals.

178. Gratz, R. R. Children's responses to emergency room care: An exploratory study of personal, situational, and parental variables (Doctoral dissertation, University of Wisconsin, 1977). Dissertation Abstracts International, 1978, 38(12-B), 5834-5835.

This study investigates children's responses in, and to, an important yet long-neglected area of pediatric medical care--the emergency room (ER). Of the personal variables studied, only age was found to be significantly related to the type of stress response exhibited. The verbalization categories of fears, curiosity, and concern about the immediate future were also found to be significant with respect to stress response: children verbalizing fears had protest scores significantly higher than those who did not; protest scores for children who expressed either curiosity or future concerns were found to be lower than those who did not verbalize these categories. For the situational variables, it was found that it is not the degree of injury or amount of time spent in the facility, but rather the general ER experience which probably precipitates the stress response. Parents' presence or proximity was not found to significantly affect the child's response, but parental responses of quieting and personal guilt were significantly related to the child's protest score.

179. Green, A. P. Meeting the needs of a child in hospital. Nursing Times, 1970, 66(7), 210-212.

In recent years much attention has been given to the experiences of small children in hospital. This article describes the aims of the hospital staff at the Royal Victoria Infirmary, Newcastle-upon-Tyne, which are to subject a child to the minimum amount of mental trauma and upset, and make his stay in hospital, whether short or long, a period during which his ordinary mental development continues and he is kept as comfortable, happy and occupied as possible. Visiting policies, play therapy, and the advantages of a Playroom are discussed.

180. Green, C. S. Larry thought puppet-play "childish": But it helped him face his fears. Nursing, 1975, 5(3), 30-33.

Play, as a natural developmental task, is the serious business of childhood. It should not be suspended just because a child is hospitalized. This article describes the development of a nondirective therapeutic play technique, puppet play, that would enable nurses to help a sick child get the most benefits out of play. A nurse's interaction with an eight-year-old boy hospitalized for nephropathy and progressive renal failure using this play technique is described.

181. Green, D. E. The hospitalisation of children. New Zealand Medical Journal, 1979, 89(635), 352-354.

This article outlines certain problems that are likely to occur among hospitalized children: (1) separation effects; (2) interpretation of illness as punishment; and (3) experiences of pain. The author discusses how various professional staff (nurses, play therapists, physicians, etc.) can help the child and his family to cope with these factors through the use of: (1) play therapy; (2) increased visitation; (3) limit setting by staff; (4) prior preparation of the child; and (5) co-operation between staff and parent.

182. Green, M., & Green J. G. The parent care pavilion. Children Today, 1977, 6(5), 5-8, 36.

The Parent Care Pavilion at the James Whitcomb Riley Hospital for Children in Indianapolis is described in this article. The Pavilion, with 12 parent care rooms, opened at the hospital in 1971. Each room has a bed for the child, a single or twin beds for the parent or parents, and a bath and shower. The Pavilion also has a large play-dining area, a parents' lounge, a nursing station and a laundry room. The unit is staffed with a head nurse, two full-time registered nurses and a ward clerk, all enthusiastic proponents of the concepts embodied in the parent care unit. One of the most impressive benefits of the Pavilion has been total elimination of the psychological trauma of hospitalization. In large part, this is attributable to the mothers, who feel welcome and effective and who can participate actively in the preparation and care of their children, answering their questions and helping to personalize their care.

183. Greenberg, L. W., & Rice, H. W. A pediatric-child-psychiatry liaison program in a community hospital. Journal of Medical Education, 1980, 55(2), 112-119.

In this paper the authors describe an innovative pediatric and child psychiatry liaison program in a community hospital. The primary focus of the program has been on the identification of normal and abnormal development of the hospitalized child and his family members, none of whom has obvious psychopathology. It has been directed toward and well received by medical students, pediatric residents, and paramedical personnel involved in pediatric hospital care and has increased the medical team's awareness of and sensitivities to patient and family needs.

184. Griffiths, S. S. Body image concerns of a four year old boy with meningitis. Maternal-Child Nursing Journal, 1980, 9(2), 127-136.

This paper describes the impact of hospitalization, illness, and pain on the body image of a four year old child hospitalized with meningitis. Billy's stage of cognitive and psychosexual development, family situation, and illness influenced his developing body image and response to hospitalization. He demonstrated heightened sensitivity and vulnerability of his body in relation to boundaries, sensation, and size. Through the expression of these bodily concerns, Billy was able to better cope with intrusive procedures within a threatening hospital environment.

185. Gross, C., Hedenkamp, E., Lovelace, B., & Meissner, A. M. Preparation of children for cardiac surgery using a team approach: How the services support the cardiologist. Journal of the Association for the Care of Children in Hospitals, 1976, 4(3), 12-16.

The recognition of the need of children to be well prepared for hospitalization has prompted hospitals to provide various kinds of orientation. Stanford University Hospital has employed the team approach for the preparation of children who are about to have cardiac surgery. It is unique in that, both in its inception and implementation, it has involved a team approach. The team consists of cardiologists, surgeons, play therapist, social worker, and pediatric and intensive care nurses who consider preparation a priority item. The team philosophy is that preparation is sequential. Each step requires preparation before it occurs to help minimize trauma and make hospitalization as constructive an experience as possible. This involves honesty about what will happen, the opportunity for the children to work through their experiences in play, the acknowledgment of individual feelings and reactions, and provides continuity of care by familiar core team members.

186. Gruppo, P. A. Helping the hospitalized child. Part I. Journal of Practical Nursing, 1977, 25(5), 14-17.

This article discusses the traumatic effects of hospitalization upon young children including separation from parents, fears about illness and treatment, and placement in a strange and unusual environment. The author outlines some of the responses children may demonstrate under these circumstances and how to deal with them. Discussion is also given to the role of the parent, how to effectively interview parents, and how they can be integrated into the hospital program to help the child.

187. Gruppo, P. A. Helping the hospitalized child. Part II. The older child. Journal of Practical Nursing, 1977, 27(6), 24-26.

This article describes the issues which hospitalized adolescents may have to deal with including adapting to a new environment, overcoming threats to self-image, and maintaining self-esteem. The author discusses several techniques including therapeutic play and body outline tools to help the adolescent with these issues. Case studies are presented to support the author's points.

188. Guerin, L. S. Hospitalization as a positive experience for poverty children: Observations on children from low-income, multi-problem families. Clinical Pediatrics, 1977, 16(6), 509-513.

The author points out the need for a clearer understanding of what the hospital means to poor children and their families. It is tragic comment on our society when a hospital becomes a refuge for many children from low-income, multi-problem families. It is even more tragic that the positive impact cannot be maintained or supported because of the complexity and rigidity of the culture in which these children live. Community agencies are ineffective for the most part because of the enormity and depth of the problems they must deal with. Money and resources are not available to provide extensive supportive and rehabilitative services in poverty areas, so real growth and change cannot occur. It is the nature of poverty life, with its corrosive effects on the body, mind and spirit, that lies at the heart of the problems discussed in this paper.

189. Hadley, B. J. Critique of "The effects of hospitalization on the coping behaviors of children." In M. V. Batey (Ed.), Communicating nursing research. Boulder, Colorado: Western Interstate Commission for Higher Eduation, 1972, 127-131.

This paper presents a critique of "The effects of hospitalization on the coping behaviors of children" by M. H. Rose. The author feels that Dr. Rose's presentation would have been enhanced by a more systematic conceptual and theoretical development of the hypotheses, particularly in terms of the conceptual framework for the theoretical premises. Further, the variables inherent in the sample seem, to the critic, to be totally uncontrollable, and questions are raised regarding the approach to the gathering of the data.

190. Hagemann, V. P. Night sleep of children in a hospital (Doctoral dissertation, University of Pittsburgh, 1978). Dissertation Abstracts International, 1979, 39(8-B), 3762.

The problem examined in this study was sleep duration and disruption of young children during the night following admission to a hospital. Thirty-four children between the ages of three and eight were observed in their hospital room throughout the sleep period. All of the children were admitted for either diagnostic evaluation or elective surgery. The children obtained less sleep during the first night in the hospital than is typical of the same age children at home. The duration of the children's sleep was affected by times of sleep onset, sleep termination, and the duration of sleep disruptions. Lateness of the time the children went to sleep significantly reduced their total amount of sleep. The delay in sleep onset resulted from hospital routines and disturbances, physical discomfort of the children, or the children's resistance to going to sleep. Early sleep termination affected the children's duration of sleep to a lesser extent than sleep onset. Many children admitted for elective surgery remained awake following the routine early morning pre-operative bath. Sleep disruptions further reduced the children's duration of sleep. The longest sleep disruptions occurred most often among those children with a medical problem who were admitted with symptoms of discomfort. These longer, less frequent disruptions, occurred early in the sleep period from physiological distress or non-specific causes. The most frequent disruptions occurred when the nursing staff awakened the children to obtain their temperature, pulse, and respiration. These disruptions were of short duration. The frequency and distribution of sleep disruptions prevented all of the children from having adequate periods of uninterrupted sleep. The preschool children experienced more sleep loss than the early school age children. Neither the physical condition of the children, their sex, nor the children's previous hospital experience or the presence of their mothers had any relationship to the duration of the children's sleep. Children with symptoms of discomfort, common among those children with a previous hospital experience, medical condition and whose mothers were present, accounted for the large number of long sleep disruptions originating with the children.

191. Haka-Ikse, K., & Leeuwen, J. V. Care of the long-term hospitalized infant. Clinical Pediatrics, 1976, 15(7), 585-588.

A clinical pilot project was carried on in an infant ward, aiming to define alternate plans for care of the long-term hospitalized young child. Impressionistic evaluations of the results of the project were encouraging in the multidisciplinary team approach. Focusing on the total needs of the child and his family seems to be helpful in mitigating the ill effects of prolonged hospitalization. The project's approach was based on common sense, developmental principles, and on a child advocacy stance whereupon not providing adequate preventive child care can be equated with neglect. It is felt that establishment of comparable multidisciplinary teams as the one described or routine provision of auxillary child care consultation to all infant wards will be a step ahead in preventing developmental difficulties stemming from long-term hospitalization.

192. Haliburton, J. Volunteer help for the frightened child. Dimensions in Health Service, 1979, 56(5), 39.

This article describes a volunteer group of women for which a core service was orientation to hospital for children. The steps taken to set up and maintain the program are discussed. Although a formal evaluation study has not been carried out, the nurses on the children's ward where the program was instituted state that children who have had the orientation provided by the volunteer group settle into the hospital routine with less trauma and seem to recover more quickly from surgery than children who have not had any orientation.

193. Hall, D. J. Social relations and innovation: Changing the state of play in hospitals. London: Routledge & Kegan Paul, 1977.

This book presents data on a situation of planned change in hospital wards. The areas addressed can be seen, like widening circles, to involve three topics of increasing diffusion. The first relates to changes in children's behaviour, the second to relationships between staff and playleaders, and the third to the responsiveness of the hospital as an organization, through the values declared by the protagonists, to change and reform. Children and change are the dual themes of the first part, in which the author tries to outline some of the major arguments drawn from studies of children and of organizations with reference to the hospital observations. Part two has as its theme observations in children's wards. Part three discusses power, negotiation and the maintenance of order.

194. Hall, D. J. Bedside blues: The impact of social research on the hospital treatment of sick children. Journal of Advanced Nursing, 1978, 3(1), 25-36.

The development of changes in the treatment of the welfare of children in hospital has a long history and some resistances are still to be found to unrestricted parental visiting and the introduction of play facilities. This paper surveys the contribution of social research to the care of children and argues against the uncritical adoption of "rule of thumb" procedures. Instead, a closer cooperation between research and practice is proposed to help overcome the problems of implementing change in hospitals.

195. Hall, D. J. On calling for order: Aspects of the organization of patient care. In D. Hall and M. Stacey (Eds.), Beyond separation: Further studies of children in hospital. London: Routledge & Kegan Paul, Ltd., 1979, 155-178.

The purpose of this chapter is to explore the world of the hospital and to suggest that it has not been paid sufficient attention as a special case of social relationships which involve and affect children's activities. The argument is made that consideration of children's response to hospital cannot be divorced from consideration of that environment as a social system, constituted and reconstituted by the pattern of encounters among participants. In terms of changes to hospital procedures, since the gap between the social situation of the child in home and in hospital is seen as one contribution to the discontinuity of hospital stay, it is suggested that solutions such as play schemes may be usefully applied. Additionally, it is recommended that much more attention should be paid to the reduction of uncertainty and ambiguity for children on the ward and that parents should be given greater information about hospital procedures and actively involved in the care of their children in hospital. All grades of staff should be chosen with regard for their understanding and sympathy for children, and greater training should be given to staff in the emotional and educational needs of children.

196. Hall, D. J., & Stacey, M. (Eds.). Beyond separation: Further studies of children in hospital. London: Routledge & Kegan Paul, Ltd., 1979.

While the editors of this volume acknowledge a debt to the studies which first demonstrated the thesis of maternal deprivation (particularly the studies of Bowlby and the Robertsons), the theme of this volume is that just as theories of separation moved beyond a medical model of treatment of disease to show the importance of the child's attachment to his social world, so now we must move beyond separation if we are to recognize the full complexity of children's response to hospital, and having recognized the complexity, to propose and test ways of resolving the problems encountered.

197. Hall, M. D. The child psychologist in an ecologically-oriented comprehensive health care program. Journal of Pediatric Psychology, 1976, 1(4), 12-13.

From the point of view of the mental health services and from the disciplinary perspective of child psychology, this author explores two of the activities in which mental health professionals have been involved at the Children's Health Center of Minneapolis. One activity relates to a group of staff nurses whose responsibility for creating and maintaining a sound emotional climate conducive to healing in a ward reserved for seriously and chronically ill older children carries with it the need for psychological support. The second activity relates to mental health consultations with the broader array of caregivers: parents, teachers, day-care personnel, all of those who determine the quality of the child's life space.

198. Hames, C. C., & Ingham, M. The colorful creatures of continuous child care. MCN: American Journal of Maternal Child Nursing, 1977, 2(6), 385-386.

Hospitalization is potentially a most traumatic experience for a child. Changes occur in almost every aspect of his life: his health is at a lower-than-usual level; he suffers the loss of significant people and objects, bombardment by strange people, and pronounced changes in physical surroundings and daily routine. These stresses combined may create more detrimental and lasting disturbances of the child's personality than the physical problems that led to his hospitalization. A simple and effective way of providing the environmental continuity the child needs and thus minimizing stress for him is described. Upon admission to the South County Hospital in Wakefield, Rhode Island, each child receives a large, bright, construction-paper cutout of a familiar animal or story character on which is noted unique behaviors or characteristics of the child. These characteristics and behaviors have been gleaned from admission history and parents' suggestions, and provide the staff with information which allows them to give more spontaneous, individualized care.

199. Hardgrove, C. B. Working with parents on the pediatric unit. Pediatric Annals, 1972, 1(3), 44-62.

During the past three decades, a growing body of research has shown the importance of meeting the emotional and developmental needs of young children during hospitalization. It is easier than one would think to humanize the pediatric ward. Children need parents; and parents need support. Opening the environment to families fosters a people-centered spirit which is natural and calming, where everyone uses a fuller self and where there is greater mutual trust. Opportunities to observe facilitate learning; parents learn from staff memebers who, in turn, gain a truer picture of parental strengths and weaknesses. Earlier dismissal is possible because staff members know what the parent can manage. Although we have a long way to go to fully exploit the potential of hospitals and the families they serve, the author concludes that rooming-in programs are a giant step in this direction. The home-like pediatric unit is one way the institution can help by strengthening the family.

200. Hardgrove, C. B. Living-in accommodations and practices for parents in hospital pediatric units: An update. Journal of the Association for the Care of Children in Hospitals, 1975, 4(1), 24-26.

In less than a decade, the concept of hospital rooming-in has gained considerable attention and acceptance. Parent organizations, pediatricians, child psychologists, pediatric nurses and family health care planners have provided abundant evidence that traumatic emotional effect on children, especially young children, resulted from their hospital experience, the primary cause being the separation from their parents. This article describes a study undertaken to survey the quantity and adequacy of overnight facilities for parents (or surrogates) of children between the ages of six months and five years. The study reinforces the need for improved public and professional understanding of both the advantages of living-in programs and the weaknesses that exist in current programs. While significant progress in the growth of such services is a cause for rejoicing, the focus of professionals and parent groups must now center upon improving the services available, strengthening parent-staff relations and inservice training programs, and in providing a comprehensive range of informational services to parents facing the stressful prospect of a hospitalized child.

201. Hardgrove, C. B. Emotional innoculation: The 3 R's of preparation. Journal of the Association for the Care of Children in Hospitals, 1977, 5(4), 17-19.

Therapeutic play for children in hospitals includes those activities that help the child marshall resources to make the new experience tolerable, perhaps even educational. The three R's that contribute to successful preparation are: rehearsal, reassurance, and recapitulation. Each phase is enhanced by the presence of a trusted adult. Without such support, even the finest preparation may fall short, because an unsupported child spends so much energy orientating to the foreign situation that there is little energy left to obtain information regardless of quality.

202. Hardgrove, C. B. Children respond to therapeuric art. Hospitals, 1980, 54(8), 67-69.

Children in the hospital have concerns that accompany their developmental state, their cognitive skills, their perception of reality, and their ability to distinguish fact from fantasy. Hospital decor should help them to cope with rather than add to their stress. Decor that includes the familiar, the interesting, and the reassuring encourages their participation in living and reminds them of the world beyond the hospital. Too much cuteness, distorted reality, incomplete or broken figures, and animals or fantasy creatures can be potentially frightening to younger chidlren and insulting to older children. An important element of the child advocate's job is to ensure that the atmosphere is therapeutic as well as cheerful through activitiy, decoration, and design.

203. Hardgrove, C. B., & Dawson, R. B. Parents and children in the hospital: The family's role in pediatrics. Boston: Little, Brown and Company, 1972.

During the last three decades, an increasing body of

research has indicated the importance of meeting the emotional and developmental needs of young children during times of hospitalization. Today, there is ample evidence that, while many children in American hospitals receive high-quality technical care, their social and emotional development may be permanently damaged because little attention is paid to their reactions to separation from the family. The study described in this book was undertaken because of an awareness of the growing concern of many professional people with the total development of the hospitalized child, because of the investigators' interest in the well-being of preschool children in particular, and because of the need for more widespread understanding of children's reactions to hospitalization. A sampling of hospitals currently carrying out innovative programs for meeting the needs of both the hospitalized child and his family were selected. The programs are described in a way intended to show, as accurately as possible, what they are really like from day to day, what the tone of the units conveys to the family and the child, and what the professional staff says and feels about such programs.

204. Hardgrove, C. B., & Rutledge, A. Parenting during hospitalization. American Journal of Nursing, 1975, 75(5), 836-838.

Parents may need coaching and support, but they are the child's best hope for making hospitalization a useful experience. The short-term stay and the first days of a long admission are most important times for parents to live in the hospital to maintain the home ties. With parents present, the child can continue learning and growing throughout the hospital experience. This article describes a program in effect at Moffett Hospital in San Francisco concerned with parental visiting of hospitalized children. Parents are invited to stay on the pediatric unit despite the lack of planned accommodations. Thus, parenting continues by night as well as by day. The message of welcome permeates the ward climate, touching even the children whose parents do not stay. The presence of parents has made it possible for the nurses to go on rounds with doctors. They can report knowledgeably to the parents about the child's medical management, and the interaction between parents and nurses reduces some of the anxious questioning that was formerly inevitable and time-consuming.

205. Harding, V. The growth of hospital play schemes in Britain. Journal of the Association for the Care of Children in Hospitals, 1976, 4(4), 16-18.

This article discusses the current situation of hospital play in the United Kingdom. The history of hospital play schemes in Britain is similar to that in the USA and Canada. These grew out of informal provision of play for young children in pediatric wards into the professionally run play programs as they are known today. In the United Kingdom this professional involvement developed from the participation and liaison of organizations such as the Pre-School Playgroups Association (PPA), Save the Children Fund (SCF), and the National Association for the Welfare of Children in Hospital (NAWCH). Each of these organizations has a wide interest in child care apart from the provision of such play programs, but each was able to contribute trained, experienced, and motivated play staff for employment and inservice training.

206. Harding, V. The importance of play. Nursing Mirror, 1977, 144 (3), 46-48.

Play is an essential part of learning to live and children play according to age and stage of development. Through play a child experiences new situations, communicates feelings and ideas, copes with frustrations or frightening events, develops skills, prepares himself for his adult role and investigates his identity. Because of the recognized importance of play, it is now known to have an important role in the care of children in hospital. By bringing play into the pediatric ward, part of the child's normal way of life is brought into the seemingly alien atmosphere of hospital. The roles of play specialists, play schemes, and play staff and family groups are described and examined. Through communication, a sharing of ideas, and a desire to learn together, the members of a pediatric team can help to make the child's stay in hospital a positive gain for the whole family.

207. Harrison, S. P. A matter of routine: Relationships between temporary disablement patterns of stress and type of care. Nursing Times, 1974, 70(37), 65-68.

In certain disabling conditions in children, the trend towards shorter stay in hospital may create a new set of social problems for parents. The concepts of stress and crisis are defined and three stress-provoking factors for parents are identified. The factors are associated with patterns of communication, finance and absence of supportive services, and the differences between parents and children who receive long-term and short-term hospital care for a temporarily disabling condition. The type and frequency of referrals between hospital and community-based staff for children providing long-term treatment are investigated, and recommendations made for the type and timing of planned intervention to reduce stress.

208. Harvey, S., & Hales-Tooke, A. (Eds.). Play in hospital. London: Faber and Faber, 1972.

In 1966 the UK National Committee of the World Organization for Early Childhood Education (OMEP) sponsored a working part to consider the value of play for children in hospital. As a result, this report was produced by people actively concerned with the well-being of children in hospital. This study included the provision of play for children of all ages from infancy to adolescence who were treated in children's wards. It was unanimously agreed that if children in hospital were to have a new deal, unrestricted visiting and generous arrangements for play must be organized. Play schemes have since been introduced into many hospitals and the authors hope the experience which has been gained and which is recorded in this book will be useful for those who promote play or who specialize in providing play for sick and handicapped children in any setting.

209. Haslett, N. Environmental contributions to the care of hospitalized children. Journal of the Association for the Care of Children in Hospitals, 1976, 5(2), 14-17.

Three and one-half to four million children under 15 years of age are hospitalized each year. One-third of all children will have spent some time in hospitals by the time they reach adulthood. This article discusses the concept of normalization of children's experience in the hospital. Suggestions are made which bear on the planning of hospital environments that will result in as normal an experience as possible for the children involved. Most of the measures discussed cost little financially, and can be made possible by lowering the threshold of awareness of children's differences from adults and appreciation of the role the environment plays in affecting the emotional life of those in it.

210. Haver, K. Reactions of a three-year-old boy to partial immobilization. Maternal-Child Nursing Journal, 1974, 3(2), 133-138.

The author describes the behaviors and coping responses of a young boy to partial immobilization caused by a broken clavicle. Outside the hospital, the boy invested a great deal of energy and concentration in learning to master his bodily functions and muscular abilities within the limitations of his immobility. After the first week these efforts toward mastery were successful and gave him a new and greater sense of pride and accomplishment. However, in the unfamiliar setting of the hospital, Michael was unable to cope successfully. He collapsed into periods of crying and depression, became hyperactive or withdrawn, and even lost control to the point of being unable to function without the help of a trusted parent. He had had no previous experience with doctors or hospitals, and therefore he knew no feeling of pride or success in this area. Some of the other reasons for Michael's initially poor adjustment to hospitalization and some of the steps taken to ameliorate the problems are further discussed.

211. Hennessey, J. A. Hospitalized toddlers' responses to mothers' tape recordings during brief separations (Doctoral dissertation, University of Pittsburgh, 1974). Dissertation Abstracts International, 1974, 35(4-B), 1766-1767.

This study described hospitalized toddlers' responses to mothers' tape recordings during brief separations. Six girls and four boys, ranging in age from seventeen to thirty months, comprised the sample. The children were hospitalized for a variety of surgical and medical reasons. The length of hospitalization varied from three to fourteen days. During twenty-four of the twenty-eight sessions, the child listened to the complete recording. However, the child fell asleep or showed signs of drowsiness at the completion of the story in fifteen sessions. Three times a child fell asleep prior to the completion of the recording. Indicators of pleasure occurred almost two times for every one occurrence of displeasure. The children indulged in self-comforting behavior such as stroking and sucking in response to the story. They followed the reading, pointing to pictures and repeating words or phrases used by the mother. The soothing effect of the recording suggests a tactile quality in the mother's voice which lifted the child temporarily out of his loneliness and seemed to reunite him with his mother. It seemed evident that hearing the mother's voice evoked the image of the mother in her absence.

212. Hennessey, J. A. Hospitalized toddlers' responses to mothers' tape recordings during brief separations. <u>Maternal-Child Nursing Journal</u>, 1976, <u>5</u>(2), 69-91.

This article describes hospitalized toddlers' responses to mothers' tape recordings during brief separations. Six girls and four boys, ranging in age from 17 to 30 months, comprised the sample. Subjects were hospitalized for a variety of surgical and medical reasons, and their length of hospitalization varied from three to 24 days. Subjects' verbal and nonverbal behaviors were observed while they listened to tape recordings of their mothers reading a story in which two major themes predominated: mother-child interaction, and separation. Twenty-eight sessions were conducted. Subjects fell asleep or showed signs of drowsiness upon completion of the story in 15 of the sessions. Indicators of pleasure occurred almost twice as often as those of displeasure. Subjects engaged in self-comforting behaviors such as stroking and sucking in response to the story; they followed the reading, pointing to pictures and repeating words or phrases used by the mother. The soothing effect of the recording suggests a tactile quality in the mother's voice which lifted the subject temporarily out of loneliness and reunited him or her with the mother. It seemed evident that hearing the mother's voice evoked the image of the mother in her absence.

213. Hersh, S. P. A perspective on behavioral medicine and pediatric psychology. Journal of Pediatric Psychology, 1976, 1(4), 3-4.

During the past 200 years and continuing over the last decade, huge strides have been made toward improvement in the education, welfare, and health of children. These strides include increased knowledge about the behavior and needs of children in hospitals. However, much remains to be done, and pediatric psychology and behavioral medicine have roles to play in future advances in these fields. This article reviews the history of child care and makes recommendations for areas requiring further development.

214. Hester, N. K. O. The preoperational child's reaction to immunization. Nursing Research, 1979, 28(4), 250-255.

Forty-four children, aged four to seven, who attended two midwestern metropolitan immunization clinics were studied in an attempt to ascertain their responses to a painful stimulus and to observe correlations between their behavioral responses and their subjective ratings of the experience. The children were screened with three tests--two Piaget tests for the preoperational stage of development and the Denver Development Screening Test for normal development. The children were observed for verbal, vocal, facial, and motor behavior during diphtheria-pertussis-tetanus or diphtheria-tetanus injections. The children then rated the extent of pain during the injection by responding to two instruments, a modification of Eland's Projective Tool and Hester's Poker Chip Tool. Each behavior category was correlated with the pain rating. Significant positive correlations were found for verbal and vocal behaviors while significant negative correlations were found for facial and motor behaviors.

215. Hill, C. J. S. The mother on the pediatric ward: Insider or outlawed? Pediatric Nursing, 1978, 4(5), 26-29.

The results of the author's study reinforce the idea that mothers of hospitalized children do wish to care for their children and that the amount of participation varies from mother to mother. Assisting the mother in caring for her child involves careful planning on the part of the nurse and the mother together, beginning at the time of admission and continuing on through the child's discharge. In this way the mother can become a member of the team caring for her child rather than remaining a passive onlooker.

216. Hilt, N. E. Pride, prejudice, and parents: A personal philosophy of pediatric parental care. Pediatric Nursing, 1976, 2(3), 32-35.

This article identifies five common pitfalls for nursing staff that may interfere with what could otherwise be accomplished with parents and patients. To eliminate these common pitfalls, each pediatric nurse must be challenged to establish, acknowledge and implement a philosophy of parental care which will be conducive to the child's well-being, permit individuality and promote a higher standard of family-centered care. The effects of these various pitfalls and how to avoid them are detailed by the author.

217. Hinz, E. Coping strategies of a two year old girl hospitalized for cardiac catheterization. Maternal-Child Nursing Journal, 1980, 9 (1), 1-6.

This article describes the experiences and the unique coping strategies of one toddler, Rachel, who was hospitalized for cardiac catheterization and evaluation of a congenital heart defect that had been detected in early infancy. Rachel experienced stress because of separation from her parents and threats to her autonomy during her brief hospitalization. A consistent relationship with the nurse seemed to be helpful in lessening the potential trauma of her experiences. This relationship was supportive of Rachel's coping devices which included the utilization of impressive verbal skills, regression, and solitary play.

218. Hoffman, P. The use of guitar and singing in a Child Life Program. Journal of the Association for the Care of Children in Hospitals, 1975, 4(1), 45-47.

When therapists and social workers write case studies of their work with children, they are most fortunate in that their therapeutic milieu is for the most part a verbal one, and therefore vocabulary exists for describing their experiences. With music, however, it becomes most difficult to delineate exactly what it is that makes it so often efficacious when helping children cope with the anxieties of hospitalization. Experiences with music in a Child Life Program show that this enigmatic quality of music not only creates a pleasurable atmosphere conducive to relaxation and the warding off of anxiety, but also contributes to increased verbalization of feelings on the part of many children. This article explores some theoretical reasons for this observed enigmatic quality of music, and also illustrates its practical application in a Child Life Program.

219. Hofmann, A. D. The hospitalized adolescent. Pediatric Annals, 1973, 2(6), 49-64.

This article describes the special case of the hospitalized adolescent. Although most adolescent patients are enthusiastic and cooperative participants in their health care, at times physicians and nurses become frustrated and even angered by some youthful patients, and the hospital staff often experiences anxiety on contemplating caring for young people. Hospital personnel often fail to take into account the adolescent's unique maturational needs, and engage in efforts to either impose parental authoritarianism or appeal to rational maturity. Both approaches are often doomed to failure; the first because it creates a power struggle no one can win, and the second because it presupposes a developmental level the young person does not possess. Knowledge of adolescent development and of human responses to stress helps in understanding how young people may be affected by serious illness or hospitalization, how they may respond to them, and how they may most effectively be helped. At the very least, the application of such knowledge will promote patient cooperation. Optimally, it will enhance positive responses, inhibit maladaptive behavior, and assist the youth to cope constructively with his or her disability.

220. Hofmann, A. D. The impact of illness in adolescence and coping behavior. Acta Paediatrica Scandinavica, 1975, Supplement #256, 29-33.

The emotional impact of serious illness or injury bears just as much potential for being disabling to an adolescent as does the condition itself. It is also these concerns and the possibilities for difficult behavior on the part of teenagers on the ward which frequently cause staff members to feel at a loss when caring for this reputedly difficult age group. But if one carefully examines the specific developmental stresses of illness and the various coping mechanisms by which the youth may counter them, a logical management approach emerges. To a large degree this approach depends on compensation, intellectualization, displacement and constructive denial but also recognizes that destructive denial, regression and projection do normally and naturally occur at various points in the course of illness and hospitalization and that panic and acting out may also readily occur, but less frequently. The deterence of the more deleterious responses and promotion of the more felicitous depends on a ward setting which provides for the adolescent's growing need for independence and self-determination; for continued reassurance about body image integrity, for resumption of mastery and control; and for the maintenance or restoration of his sense of self-worth. These goals are achieved by encouraging the youth to be an active partner in his own care; to share in decisions made about his condition; to pursue just as much independent self-management as he can; to actively engage in establishing a peer group with other adolescents in the ward; to continue with his education, socialization, personal interests and outside peer contacts as much as possible; and to feel that the staff respects his dignity and privacy, likes him as a person and appreciates the courage and effort with which he is facing a difficult time.

221. Hofmann, A. D., & Becker, R. D. Psychotherapeutic approaches to the physically ill adolescent. International Journal of Child Psychotherapy, 1973, 2(4), 492-511.

The authors present a selective review of the psychological reactions of adolescents to illness and hospitalization. A critical examination of defensive and coping mechanisms invoked to combat anxiety is systematically discussed. Therapeutic guidelines are suggested which will encourage those preexisting and naturally occurring healthy strategies essential to satisfactory readjustment after hospitalization. The characteristic responses of adolescents to medical or surgical crises are reviewed. The importance of recognizing the anxieties actuated by illness, surgery, or hospitalization among this age group, is stressed. The role of the consulting psychiatrist or psychologist on the medical unit is considered.

222. Hofmann, A. D., Becker, R. D., & Gabriel, H. P. The hospitalized adolescent: A guide to managing the ill and injured youth. New York: The Free Press, 1976.

The goal of this book is to promote understanding of the full scope of adolescent growth and development and the effects of illness, injury, and hospitalization thereon, encouraging the implementation of a health care system that will optimally promote the teen-ager's return to his normal business of growing up and realizing the full potential of his life. Part I is a theoretical examination of those developmental issues upon which the authors' management techniques are based. Part II offers a set of basic management principles applicable to all patients and begins by looking at the mechanics of organizing and staffing the ward itself. Part III responds to a number of particularly difficult and thorny situations that inevitably crop up on every adolescent ward from time to time and pose singular stress to all concerned. There has been an attempt to present the material in an interdisciplinary way and to make it relevant to the concerns of all professionals who are responsible for hospitalized adolescents in any capacity.

223. Holmes, S. The use of control by a hospitalized five year old girl. Maternal-Child Nursing Journal, 1976, 5(3), 189-196.

The author describes the controlling behaviors manifested by a five-year-old during her hospitalization for back surgery due to malformed lower vertebrae. A complication of her hospitalization was dysuria characterized by frequency of and difficulty in voiding. The subject was discharged on the ninth day after surgery, 16 days after admission to the hospital. The subject's use of control is related to the two main concerns of the preschool years: body function, and body integrity. Her controlling behaviors were expressed through verbal commands, play and fantasy, and physical maintenance of self-control by holding in.

224. Hood, C. Children abandoned in long-stay hospitals. Child: Care, Health and Development, 1976, 2, 239-250.

This study investigates some aspects of the problems of abandonment of children in hospital, employing a sample of sixty-eight children from six selected hospitals, who meet a given definition of abandonment. Almost a fifth of the total population of children in the hospitals studied meet this definition; about a third of the sample are abandoned early in their lives, and for the remainder, admission itself appears to be a factor in abandonment.

225. Hott, J. Rx: Play PRN in pediatric nursing. Nursing Forum, 1970, 9(3), 288-309.

Changes in knowledge about human growth, stimulated by the behaviorists and norms of motor development, plus increased understanding through psychoanalysis of personality development, have contributed toward an altered evaluation of play and fun. This article discusses the concept of "therapeutic community" in the hospital, where play must be a part of the total service and all the people working with each child must be concerned with more than just the child's physical needs. Theories of play are examined in order to help nurses who work with children implement the concept of play as therapy.

226. Hughes, A. H., & Dudley, H. K., Jr. Mental care for children. Hospitals, 1973, 47(2), 54, 56-57.

For many years, there has been a growing concern over the number of mentally ill and emotionally disturbed children in the United States. Evidence suggests that between 10 and 12 per cent of the 50 million school-age children have moderate to severe emotional problems requiring some kind of mental health service. State mental institutions must design programs that will give young patients the opportuntiy to develop stable personalities and to become responsible citizens within the limits of their potential. In many cases, the hospitals also must ensure that young patients do not return to the sort of unstable home life that caused their problems. Nothing can be gained by sending a child who has undergone treatment back to his family unless the family environment also has changed. For this reason hospitals should initiate programs of parent training and/or counseling within their communities. Four areas of personal development included in a basic program outline initiated by many Texas state hospitals are described: (1) physical development; (2) social development; (3) emotional therapy; and (4) intellectual development.

227. Hunnisett, F. W., & Knowles, D. J. Orienting prospective patients. Hospitals, 1970, 44, 51-53.

Any children's hospital must provide not only the best possible care for its patients, but try to reduce the traumatic effects of hospitalization from which so many children suffer. Unfortunately, parents often contribute to this trauma without realizing that they do so. They feel inadequate and incapable of discussing with the child his forthcoming admission. Fear of the unknown and the horror of separation from parents cause frustration to both children and parents. The child often arrives at the hospital admitting department in a condition of mental anguish that affects not only his behavior but his convalescence. This article describes how prospective patients at a major children's hospital in Toronto are oriented to the hospital environment and prepared for their inpatient experience through a preadmission program that eases fear for the children and their parents.

228. Hunt, A. D. On the hospitalization of children: An historical approach. Pediatrics, 1974, 54(5), 542-546.

This article provides a brief history of children's hospitalization procedures and practices from the mid-eighteenth century to the present. Visiting policies, both past and present, are discussed. A modern children's hospital which provides an entire range of children's services, from preventive well-child care to the most technical and dramatic of medical and surgical manipulations is discribed. The author concludes that such a hospital, properly planned and organized, must have as its common denominator the welfare of the child. Such a concern should reflect itself in meticulous attention to detail in physical planning, design, construction, staffing, equipment, admission procedures, visiting hours, patient care, discharge planning, and outpatient management. Such effort, oriented around the needs of patients, will produce the ultimate in quality and efficiency of care.

229. Huntington, D. S. Learning from infants and families. Journal of the Association for the Care of Children in Hospitals, 1975, 4(1), 5-20.

This article outlines ways of learning from infants and their families with regard to hospitalization. Two broad themes are followed: first, fostering competence, and second, promotive and active efforts as the framework of the future. The history of infants in hospitals is discussed and the effects of hospitalization on infants is examined.

230. Hymovich, D. P. The pediatric nursing role as perceived by nursing personnel and four- to eight-year-old hospitalized children (Doctoral dissertation, University of Maryland, 1973). Dissertation Abstracts International, 1974, 34(11-B), 5534-5535.

This study was an investigation of perceptions which hospitalized four- to eight-year-old children and hospital nurses have of the pediatric nursing role. The population included selected four- to eight-year-old children (N = 41) in three metropolitan hospitals and the nursing personnel (N = 40) caring for them. Two instruments were developed for the study: The Role Perception Picture Inventory and The Role Taking Inventory. A third instrument, Least Preferred Coworker scale, was also employed. Analysis of the data failed to support Hypothesis I which states that hospitalized four- to eight-year old surgical patients perceive the nursing role as more instrumental than do nonsurgical patients of the same age. Hypothesis II, which states that nursing personnel perceive their role as more expressive than do four- to eight-year-old children, was not supported for the total sample but was supported for nurses and seven-year-old patients. Hypothesis III states that children are unable to take the perspective of nursing personnel in perceiving the nursing role. This hypothesis was supported by responses to 14 of the 16 questions. No support was found for Hypothesis IV which states there is a positive relationship between nursing style of personnel and their role perceptions. There was some tendency for person-oriented personnel (high LPC scores) to have positive correlations between LPC scores and scores on the RPPI and RTI as predicted by the hypothesis.

231. Hymovich, D. P. Parents of sick children: Their needs and tasks. Pediatric Nursing, 1976, 2(5), 9-13.

The onset of illness in a child may precipitate a family crisis. The ability of the family to recover from the stress of illness depends in large part upon the coping ability of the parents. The parents are required to accomplish three major tasks. They must be able: (1) To understand and manage their child's illness; (2) To assist their child in understanding and coping with his/her illness; and (3) To meet the needs of all family members as well as those of the ill child. For parents to master these tasks successfully, their basic needs for information, trust, guidance and support, and resources must be met. These needs are common to all parents regardless of their child's type of illness, age or therapy. The manner in which these needs are met will differ with each family. Nursing personnel and other health professionals play a valuable role in helping parents care for their ill children. To do this effectively, they need an understanding of the impact of illness on the individual and his total family.

232. Irwin, E. C., & Kovacs, A. Analysis of children's drawings and stories. Journal of the Association for the Care of Children in Hospitals, 1979, 8(2), 39-48.

This paper reports a study undertaken to determine how children react to hospitalization and surgical experiences, as manifested in the form and content of the projected data in their spontaneous stories and drawings. Involved in this descriptive study were 60 children: 30 youngsters who had been admitted for surgery to the orthopedic unit of a large metropolitan pediatric hospital and a comparison group of 30 children who had no known previous history of hospitalization. The subjects, a total of 15 boys and 15 girls in each of two groups, were matched for sex and age. All subjects were white and ranged in age from six to twelve. One finding, confirmed by both drawings and the stories, is that many children, especially boys, are fearful of surgery that often seems to represent a kind of symbolic castration. A second major finding in this study was that hospitalized youngsters seemed to try to make sense of the situation, each trying to understand the hospitalization in his/her own personal way. An unanticipated finding of the study was the hospitalized children's reactions to the nurse examiners. The children seemed to take the opportunity to use help in talking about the hospital experience, symbolically as well as directly. The study suggests that expressive activities, such as those utilized here, can be a powerful aid to children at a time of vulnerability. The responses of the children in the study indicate that they used the empathetic help of an adult that provided cathartic relief, which, in turn, reduced stress and aided in the coping process.

233. Irwin, E. C., & McWilliams, B. J. Play therapy for children with cleft palates. *Children Today*, 1974, *3*(3), 18-22.

The results of recent research studies of young children with cleft palates suggest that these children show some deficiency in the use of expressive language. Since these deficits were found regardless of the children's speech proficiency, there is speculation that part of the problem may relate to the child's lack of desire to communicate. This article describes a creative play program to provide language stimulation for preschool children with cleft palates which utilized creative dramatics, a group activity which places a high value on verbal skills and group interaction, as an approach. The dramatic play situation provides rich opportunities for observing and assessing spontaneous speech, play and interaction in a real-life situation, as well as offering many opportunities for successful communication experiences on the child's own level. It may also be viewed as a behavior modification technique. Observers rated the extent to which a child used pantomime, the amount and appropriateness of his speech, and the nature and quality of his role-playing skills. Significant increases in all three areas were found during the second three-month period of this study. The observers' narrative and verbatim accounts also indicate that the children's communication skills improved significantly during the course of the program.

234. Isler, C. The fine art of handling a hospitalized child. *RN*, 1978, *41*(3), 41-45.

When the stress of hospitalization overwhelms a youngster, the nurse is the person who usually has to deal with the consequences. The key to a disturbed child's behavior must be found if the nurse is going to help the child come to grips with what's bothering him and modify that behavior. The best place to start is with a general understanding of what makes some hospitalized children hit, scream, cling, assault, withdraw, or otherwise behave in unusual or unacceptable ways. If nurses take time to analyze a child's behavior, and if they know what to expect from children at various ages, it is easier to identify the underlying causes of his fears and explain them in language he can understand. This article pinpoints behavior problems encountered most frequently in hospitalized children at different ages, as well as measures nurses can use to encourage acceptable behavior.

235. Issner, N. The family of the hospitalized child. Nursing Clinics of North America, 1972, 7(1), 5-12.

In dealing with the hospitalized child we must be aware that he is part of a total unit, the family, regardless of its composition. Illness has an impact not only upon the patient but upon the unit as well. We must be able to recognize the implications of hospitalization for every member of the family in order to provide optimum physical and psychologic care.

236. Issner, N. Can the child be distracted from his disease? Journal of School Health, 1973, 43(7), 468-471.

A hospital regime, no matter how geared to the needs of children, is a stressful, anxiety-producing situation. Separation fears, loss of self-esteem, fear of mutilation, etc., are well known phenomena that affect toddler and teen-ager alike. Although efforts are being made at many medical centers to reduce the psychological effects of these stresses by play programs, these approaches often skirt the basic issue of a child's need to know what is going on around him, especially with regard to his physical self.

237. Jackson, D. W. The adolescent and the hospital. Pediatric Clinics of North America, 1973, 20(4), 901-910.

Hospitalization is a time of crisis no matter what the age or lifestyle of the patient may be. The discussion in this article, however, has been limited to the hospitalization of the adolescent. The discussion focuses on two points: (1) whether or not the reaction of youth to hospitalization is significantly different from that of other age groups; and (2) whether or not the care and surroundings of adolescents require modification.

238. Jackson, P. B., Bradham, R. F., & Burwell, H. K. Child care in the hospital--A parent/staff partnership. MCN: American Journal of Maternal Child Nursing, 1978, 3(2), 104-107.

This article describes a study that examined at admission parents' desires for participation in their child's care. While the limitations of size and setting in the study must be considered, for this population at least the results were very positive. Parents wanted a high degree of participation in child care and were able to do as they wished. Other nurses were encouraged to ask parents early in their child's hospitalization about their desire for participating in child care. By doing so, an opportunity for parents to continue in some semblance of their familiar role with their children can be provided, thus easing the stress on the family and promoting a continued close parent/child relationship.

239. Jacobs, R. The meaning of hospital: Denial of emotions. In D. Hall and M. Stacey (Eds.), Beyond separation: Further studies of children in hospital. London: Routledge & Kegan Paul, Ltd., 1979, 82-108.

This chapter focuses on the denial of feeling which is seen to be an important contribution to, as well as a consequence of, children's disturbance in hospital. In particular, the nature of the orthopedic hospital as a "total institution," isolated from the outside world, is emphasized, and the consequences for the type of control and socialization exerted by staff over patients is discussed. Elements of depersonalization, of treating the patient as a work-object are identified, and the treatment of illness as a matter of routine by staff is contrasted with the immediacy of illness as a crisis to the individual child (and to the parents). The most important practical implication of the study reported emphasizes the dialectical character of illness and the social institutions connected with it. Thus in order that staff may themselves provide psychosocial support in the ward situation, both to each other and to the patients, they must themselves be given such strength and succour from others within the social organization in which they work. Furthermore, for change to take place within institutions that are dominated by an ideology characterized by denial of feeling, such support must be readily available to staff. This is a necessary precondition for change in the orientation of staff, and the quality of the care given in the ward will in turn reflect and relate to these values.

240. James, V. L., Jr. Care-by-parent unit cuts costs, benefits hospitalized child. Hospital Topics, 1972, 50(9), 72-74.

The accelerating rise in hospital cost, the mounting shortage of nurses, the obvious desirability of keeping a mother and child together during a crisis situation and the necessity of teaching mothers how to care for their children's needs, have combined to make experimentation in the hospital care of children a vital necessity. The Care-by-Parent Unit at the University of Kentucky Medical Center was established in an attempt to answer to some of these problems. The Care-by-Parent Unit is specifically designed so that parents will stay with their children in the hospital and provide what care is needed by the child during the hospital stay. This article describes the operation of this special program and discusses the following advantages associated with the unit: (1) a significant reduction in the cost of hospitalization; (2) an elimination of the trauma of mother-child separation; (3) better after-hospital care because of an increase in parents' knowledge and ability; and (4) addition of another dimension of care in the teaching of medical students and house staff.

241. Jankowski, J. J. Clinical child psychiatry services on a pediatric-adolescent unit. Journal of the American Academy of Child Psychiatry, 1974, 13(1), 95-109.

In adolescence, medical illness and emotional problems are often intermeshed. The psychiatric services as described in this paper attempt to satisfy the requirements of all inpatient adolescents on the pediatric ward. This seems to be a reasonable goal for child psychiatrists who consult and collaborate in providing such services. The pediatric ward holds much promise as a resource for hospitalizing emotionally troubled adolescents. It is readily available and familiar to most pediatricians who see many in this age group. It is more acceptable to the adolescent and his family to be hospitalized on a pediatric ward rather than in an inpatient psychiatric unit. However, it should remain a pediatric ward and not be converted into a quasi-psychiatric ward. Its advantages rest in precisely the fact that it is predominantly a pediatric ward, not a psychiatric facility.

242. Jay, S. S. Pediatric intensive care: Involving parents in the care of their child. Maternal-Child Nursing Journal, 1977, 6(3), 195-204.

The trauma of hospitalization has long been attributed to fear of painful procedures and separations from parents. Nurses have long supported the rights of children and parents by encouraging rooming-in and extended visiting policies. Yet the struggle has just begun to penetrate the Pediatric Intensive Care Units. This paper has two purposes: the first is to increase nurses' awareness that the child's need for his parents is greatly increased while he is in an ICU; the second is to demonstrate how to encourage and assist parental involvement with their child in Pediatric Intensive Care Units.

243. Jeffries, P. M. Free visiting for children. Nursing Times, 1973, 69(48), 1664-1665.

This article discusses some of the traditional reasons why more liberal hospital visitation policies have not been implemented: (1) Some children's nurses use their patients as an outlet for their own frustrated maternal instincts and resent parents having free access to their children; (2) Nurses cannot undertake their duties adequately if the ward is "cluttered up"; (3) Free visiting means much more work for the nursing and medical staff; (4) Student nurses may find the added stress of constant surveillance by parents in a children's ward might well prove too great a strain; (5) Student nurses have to face managing worried parents; and (6) Others in the family will be neglected due to the absence of the parents. The author reviews what measures can be taken, particularly by the ward sister, to help reduce these problems and encourage more parent-child contact.

244. Johnson, B. H. Before hospitalization: A preparation program for the child and his family. *Children Today*, 1974, *3*(6), 18-21.

Five years ago, staff members of the Children's Hospital National Medical Center in Washington, D. C., began to act upon their realization that children and parents should receive more effective preparation for hospitalization, surgery and other experiences young patients at the hospital would have to undergo. This program is described and discussed. Through the implementation of the preadmission preparation procedures, the staff has tried to identify the common concerns children and parents feel about hospitalization and to help alleviate them in a group setting, thus meeting the critical emotional needs of children and their families while realistically utilizing the professional health team most efficiently.

245. Johnson, J. E., Kirchhoff, K. T., & Endress, M. P. Altering children's distress behavior during orthopedic cast removal. *Nursing Research*, 1975, *24*(6), 404-410.

The hypothesis tested was that discrepancy between expected and experienced physical sensations (what is felt, seen, heard, tasted, and smelled) during a threatening experience will result in distress. The subjects were 84 children, six to 11 years of age, male and female. The threatening experience was orthopedic cast removal. Tape recorded preparatory information was used to vary systematically expectations about physical sensations. The children were randomly assigned to one of three information groups: (1) sensory information which described the sensory experience during cast removal; (2)procedure information which described the steps of the experience; (3) control group which heard no tape recorded information. Nonverbal and verbal signs of distress reactions and the pulse rate were observed during cast removal. As hypothesized, the mean distress score for the sensation group differed significantly from the control group mean. The procedure group distress score mean fell between the sensation and control group means but did not differ significantly from the control group mean. The no pre-fear group distress score mean was significantly lower than the same pre-fear group mean. Mean pulse rate changes for information groups for before to during cast removal were in the same order as the distress scores, but the differences were not statistically significant.

246. Johnson, J. E., Kirchhoff, K. T., & Endress, M. P. Easing children's fright during health care procedures. MCN: American Journal of Maternal Child Nursing, 1976, 1(4), 206-210.

While it is generally recognized that children are better able to cope with frightening diagnostic and treatment procedures when they are given truthful explanations, time simply does not always allow nurses to explore all aspects of the procedure at hand with an individual child. It therefore becomes necessary to be selective, covering information which will be most helpful. This article describes a particular kind of information which benefits children more than the traditionally recommended procedural explanations.

247. Johnson, P. A. A training curriculum for Child Life workers. Journal of the Association for the Care of Children in Hospitals, 1975, 4(1), 41-42.

As Child Life programs become more widespread in pediatric inpatient and outpatient facilities, the increased importance of providing training experiences for people whose teaching and therapeutic interests involve helping children deal with the potentially traumatic effects of a hospital stay is realized. This article describes a Child Life Program at the Johns Hopkins Hospital in Baltimore, Maryland, which has as its goal assistance of education and child development students to extend their skills to include experiences with hospitalized children. This approach is seen as a valuable learning experience for all who are involved.

248. Johnson, P. A., & Stockdale, D. F. Effects of puppet therapy on palmar sweating of hospitalized children. Johns Hopkins Medical Journal, 1975, 137(1), 1-5.

This study investigated effects of a puppet presentation on anxiety levels of hospitalized children as measured by the Palmar Sweat Index (PSI). Subjects were 43 children, ages five to eight inclusive, allocated randomly to treatment and nontreatment groups. Treatment consisted of a puppet show designed to familiarize patients with hospital routines and with procedures of their operations. Four PSI measures were collected from each subject, and average difference scores of individuals among all measures were compared. Analyses of variance were used to test mean differences with data categorized by treatment, by sex, and by interaction of sex and treatment. The treatment was associated with a significant reduction in anxiety from the time of admission to both (1) the period immediately after the puppet show, and (2) the evening after surgery. In the interim, the measure of anxiety returned to near the level at admission.

249. Johnston, M. Toward a culture of caring: Children, their environment, and change. MCN: American Journal of Maternal Child Nursing, 1979, 4(4), 210-214.

There are several reasons that nurses must be concerned with their patients' environment. Perhaps the most important one, however, is that an individual's personal value is often conveyed by the condition of his surroundings. This article discusses how the environment of a health care setting can be a helpful adjunct to overall care of children, and how it should be given as much consideration as the various other elements of the treatment program. The author concludes that we can no longer treat children like miniature adults. Expecting children to cope with an adult world perpetuates this mistake and distorts their perceptions. An environmental program concerned with a therapeutic environment for children at Rancho Los Amigos Hospital in Downey, California, is described.

250. Johnston, M., & Salazar, M. Preadmission program for rehospitalized children. American Journal of Nursing, 1979, 79(8), 1420-1422.

The authors describe a Family Preparation Clinic at Rancho Los Amigos Hospital, designed to help staff and families prepare for impending rehospitalizations. When families arrive at the clinic, they are met by a volunteer who helps to orient the family to the hospital. Upon returning to the clinic, a nurse and social worker from the inpatient setting where the child will be cared for, conduct a family group session, beginning with an 18-minute video tape, developed at the hospital that evokes feelings and memories of prior hospital encounters. Then a history and physical examination is done by the physician and the families leave the hospital to return three days later for direct admission to the patient care area. During the initial six months of this pilot clinic, 46 children and their families participated. There have been several observable benefits: (1) Families experienced less waiting time in diagnostic departments; (2) There is less confusion about where to go for various services within the hospital and more compliance in obtaining preadmission diagnostic studies; (3) More information is exchanged in response to parental concerns; (4) Children receive time and permission to express their feelings and receive reassurance and information about medical procedures; and (5) Parents have more contact with the day-to-day caretaking members of the staff as well as an opportunity to begin trusting relationships.

251. Jolly, H. The work of the play specialists in Charing Cross Hospital, London. Journal of the Association for the Care of Children in Hospitals, 1978, 6(2), 4-10.

The author discusses the role of play specialists in helping children cope with hospitalization by (a) reducing stress and meeting needs communicated through play, (b) eliciting information from play relevant to medical treatment, and (c) making illness an opportunity for positive learning and the hospital environment less threatening. Case examples are presented to illuminate these principles.

252. Jolly, J. D. The ward granny scheme. Nursing Times, 1974, 70 (15), 537-540.

Nurses know well how distressing it can be to have to leave a crying child because there is no time to comfort him. Although patient assignment can materially reduce the number of people actively involved in the nursing care of a child, nurses cannot provide the one-to-one relationship that is needed for the mothering care of very young children in hospitals. Because of dissatisfaction with the patient assignment method of dealing with the problem of providing personal contact and continuity needed to carry the young child through the strangeness and possibly serious trauma of hospitalization, the staff of a pediatric ward initiated a program which used ward grannies to fill the function of mother substitutes for unaccompanied young children on the ward. This program is described and discussed.

253. Jolly, J. D. The grand tour. Journal of the Association for the Care of Children in Hospitals, 1975, 3(4), 3-8.

To many Americans, the "Grand Tour" must conjure up an endless succession of ancient Gothic buildings, priceless paintings and sculptures, and exposure to the rich historical culture of Europe. To this author, the opposite was true. As an English pediatric nurse, her Grand Tour was composed of traveling the breadth of the

North American continent visiting hospitals and pediatric units, studying the latest systems of child care. This report describes some of the schemes the author observed in 43 institutions.

254. Jolly, J. D. Preparing children for hospital. Nursing Times, 1976, 72(39), 1532-1533.

This article describes several Canadian and American hospitals that specialize in the progressive care of sick children. In particular, innovative work concerning the preparation of children for admission to hospital is discussed. The author believes that preparation for the child who must enter the hospital is an important advance in hospital services.

255. Jolly, J. D. Child care in North America, 2: How to be in hospital without being frightened. Nursing Times, 1977, 73(48), 1887-1888.

There do not have to be vast resources of money or space in which a child may make his hospital experience both bearable and a positive contribution to his development. Staff do need to acquaint themselves with healthy child development and the means of communication a child has at his disposal. This article discusses children's hospital care in North America, and the importance of hospitalization preparation and play therapy is emphasized.

256. Jones, L., & Wakely, C. Tell me about your picture: Insights into children's ideas about the hospital. Imprint, 1974, 21(1), 20-22, 29.

Children are busy much of the time learning about themselves and the world around them. This article describes a study undertaken to elicit children's concepts of hospitalization through drawings and subsequent interviews. The impact of hospitalization was evident in the pictures. Results are discussed.

257. Juenker, D. Child's perception of his illness. In S. Steele (Ed.), Nursing care of the child with long-term illness. New York: Appleton-Century-Crofts, 1971, 133-171.

This chapter seeks to identify and describe the factors that influence the child's perception of illness. Emphasis is placed on those factors that are most essential in planning nursing care. The child's view of the structure and function of the body is examined. The impact of hospitalization is explored, and the chapter concludes with an analysis of parental influence. It is hoped that the information which is presented will increase the nurse's awareness of the perceptual process as it relates to a child's view of illness.

258. Juenker, D. Play as a tool of the nurse. In S. Steele (Ed.), Nursing care of the child with long-term illness. New York: Appleton-Century-Crofts, 1971, 27-95.

This chapter elaborates on the subject of play from several points of view with particular attention focused on children with long-term illnesses. The meaning and value of play is described, and age factors which influence play behavior are explored. An explanation of the nurse's role in establishing an environment that is conducive to play is included along with a description of an assessment tool for identifying play needs. One section includes a delineation of the special play problems experienced by immobilized children. The chapter concludes with an examination of the nurse-parent interaction in regard to play.

259. Kakkanatt, T., & Gnus, M. A seven year old boy's control of stress during hospitalization. Maternal-Child Nursing Journal, 1980, 9(1), 49-59.

Hospitalization and surgery on the genitalia present major threats to an early latency age child's relatively weak ego. Coping with threat under such circumstances depends on the child's ability to use his own ego resources and those resources available in the environment effectively. Successful coping implies a sense of control over the stress. This article describes the case of a seven-year-old boy hospitalized for surgery involving the genitals. Selected behaviors indicative of his coping with stress of hospitalization are identified: appraisal of threat, self-assertion, and avoidance. In his mother's presence, the child appraised danger effectively and boldly protested apparent attacks.

260. Kalafatich, A. J., & Hershberger, R. W. Approaches to hospitalized teen-agers. In A. J. Kalafatich (Ed.), Approaches to the care of adolescents. New York: Appleton-Century-Crofts, 1975, 143-193.

There are many problems of, and with, hospitalized teenagers that are common to both boys and girls. There are, however, enough differences to warrant two separate case presentations which are the subject of this chapter. The first section is primarily concerned with a teenage girl who was undergoing treatment for scoliosis, a lateral curvature of the spine. The second section is concerned with male adolescents, and the case presented is a teenage boy who became a paraplegic following an auto accident. The two case studies are discussed.

261. Kaufman, R. V. Body-image changes in physically ill teen-agers. Journal of the American Academy of Child Psychiatry, 1972, 11(1), 157-170.

The relationship of body image to self representation is discussed and case material is presented to illustrate the relationship of physical illness to changes in body image. Clinical material illustrates the far-reaching effects of sickness on the children's self representations and the varying kinds of damage portrayed. The central role of visual elements in body-image construction is discussed as lending itself to this graphic symbolism and is one link between changes in physical health and changes in body image. Such data add another dimension to assessment of the effects of hospitalization as well as the role in development of physical threat or injury.

262. Kenny, T. J. The hospitalized child. Pediatric Clinics of North America, 1975, 22(3), 583-593.

Today the pediatrician must know the course of the emotional response to hospitalization just as he must know the usual course of a disease process to maximize the response to treatment. Knowledge of the psychological process puts the physician in a better position to maximize the response to treatment by fulfilling one of his major roles in the situation. These include: (1) preparing the child for the hospital experience; (2) preparing the parents to cope with the reaction of the child to the experience; (3) preparing the parents to cope with their own concerns about the hospitalization; (4) acting as an advocate for the child during his hospitalization; and (5) acting as an agent for change to improve the hospital experience.

263. Kerr, N. J. The effect of hospitalization on the developmental tasks of childhood. Nursing Forum, 1979, 18(2), 108-130.

Although hospitalization is traumatic for all age groups, there is no doubt children are the hardest hit, because separation from the mother can produce psychological disturbances that may have a lasting effect on emotional well-being. Since the child's developmental level will influence the meaning separation has for him, this article examines the child's response to hospitalization from a developmental point of view, and considers how the trauma may affect the mother-child relationship. Some of the characteristic features, primary tasks, and major conflicts of infancy, toddlerhood, pre-school age, and latency are presented within the framework of Freudian and Eriksonian theories. Suggestions to minimize the trauma based on principles set down in studies such as the Platt Report are reviewed.

264. Klein, C. B., & Satterthwaite, M. Preparation and the hospitalized child. Journal of the Association for the Care of Children in Hospitals, 1980, 8(3), 60-63.

People who work in hospitals are endlessly bombarded with situations that are overwhelmingly tragic. The resultant psychic pain they suffer is handled either by denial and detachment, by withdrawing from the situation and requesting transfers, or even by leaving the profession. A more constructive approach would be to plan ongoing work with a highly trained consultant to gain insights and skills with which to help both the patients and staff. It then becomes clearer to staff members how and in what areas they can effectively support the patient, and which areas are truly not their responsibility. This article is written for all staff members who work with hospitalized children and gives an overview of work on the subject of preparation undertaken by a group of child life workers from Mt. Sinai Hospital, Rainbow Babies' and Children's Hospital, and The Cancer Center in Cleveland, Ohio, who meet each week with a Child Analyst at The Cleveland Center for Research in Child Development.

265. Klein, M., Roghmann, K. J., & Charney, E. The impact on the hospitalization of children. In R. J. Haggerty, K. J. Roghmann and I. B. Pless (Eds.), Child health and the community. New York: John Wiley & Sons, 1975, 253-264.

This article discusses the impact that the Rochester Neighborhood Health Center (RNHC), established in 1964, had on the hospitalization of children. The RNHC was used more by target area residents at low risk for hospitalization than by those at high risk. The admission rate of users was lower in the second year than in the first year of operation and lower than the comparison area populations. The length of hospital stays was also reduced. Health center users were admitted less for respiratory/infectious and more for surgical/elective reasons. A conservative conclusion as to the effect of the health center appears justified: for patients who were attracted to the center and became users, hospitalization rates and days declined. This is what was hoped to be the effect of the center. There remains, however, a group of children, not using the center although eligible, who continue to have high hospitalization rates.

As is true of much of the evaluation of the RNHC, hospitalization outcomes are "mixed notices."

266. Klinzing, D. G., & Klinzing, D. R. Increasing pediatric nursing staff's knowledge of child care in hospitals: A method tested, a method suggested. Journal of the Association for the Care of Children in Hospitals, 1975, 3(3), 21-22.

To determine whether the need to have medical personnel who work in pediatrics learn about the non-medical aspects of caring for hospitalized children could be met through an inservice program, a study was conducted at the Delaware Division Hospital of the Wilmington Medical Center in Wilmington, Delaware. The specific purpose of the experiemnt was to determine whether a training program could measurably improve the pediatric nursing staff's knowledge of infant stimulation, play therapy and the emotional needs of the hospitalized child and his parents.

267. Klinzing, D. G., Rothman, L., & Aukamp, D. Evaluating pediatric care programs. Journal of the Association for the Care of Children in Hospitals, 1974, 3(1), 8-10.

Today there are many changes taking place in the pediatric divisions of hospitals throughout the country. Those who have been concerned about the welfare of hospitalized children have reason to be hopeful. Some of the new facilities, programs and materials should make a considerable contribution to the quality of care given to pediatric patients. However, serious consideration must be given to the task of evaluating the newly developed pediatric programs to determine the extent to which they are meeting the needs of the hospitalized child. One such evaluation was made of the pediatric department of the Wilmington Medical Center Delaware Division Hospital in Wilmington, Delaware. The evaluation was accomplished by means of a questionnaire desinged by a faculty member and two students in consultation with several hospital staff members. The questionnaire in its final version is presented.

268. Klinzing, D. R., & Klinzing, D. G. An evaluation of video-tapes designed to communicate with children about hospitalization, surgery, and casting. Journal of the Association for the Care of Children in Hospitals, 1976, 4(3), 4-11.

Hospitalization and medical procedures can be very stressful and anxiety producing experiences for young children. Recognizing the potential of media as a technique for helping children with medical problems, Fred Rogers, the producer and star of the nationally televised children's program, "Mr. Rogers' Neighborhood," has produced three pilot video-tapes designed to prepare children for hospitalization, surgery, and having a cast applied and removed. This article describes a study undertaken to evaluate and test these tapes. The reactions of pediatric staff to the three Rogers tapes were sufficiently favorable to constitute an endorsement. It is expected that the endorsements and comments made by staff provide useful information about the strengths and limitations of the tapes and help justify the use of the tapes in experiments with children.

269. Klinzing, D. R., & Klinzing, D. G. The hospitalized child: Communication techniques for health personnel. Englewood Cliffs, New Jersey: Prentice-Hall, Inc., 1977.

This book is designed to help health care personnel become aware of how important good communication techniques are, and to learn how to use them to improve the quality of care of the hospitalized child and his family. The authors believe that hospital personnel must take responsibility for the emotional care of the hospitalized child by providing him with an environment that will effectively reduce the chances of a negative emotional response to the hospital. To achieve this the staff must know how to communicate with the child, his family, and other staff members. Several definitions and models of the communication process are explained in the first chapter, allowing the reader to familiarize himself with many factors involved in sending and receiving messages. The next section of this book examines staff and child interactions that affect a child's hospital experience. The authors give suggestions that can be followed to help make the child's first encounter in the hospital a positive experience. A chapter of this book gives suggestions for communication with the dying child and his family. Kubler-Ross's stages are outlined. The final chapter gives suggestions on how to prepare a child for a visit to the doctor's office, emergency room, or clinic.

270. Knight, R. B. Coping mechanisms used by children hospitalized for elective surgery (Doctoral dissertation, Yeshiva University, 1977). Dissertation Abstracts International, 1978, 38(9-B), 4465.

This study investigated the relationship between the effectiveness of coping mechanisms and physiological indicators of distress in children faced with the experience of hospitalization and surgery. Twenty-four children between the ages of seven and eleven were studied two weeks before surgery in the out-patient department and again during their hospital stay. Effectiveness of defenses was measured by a clinical interview and by the Rorschach. Cortisol production rates were measured by the analysis of 24-hour urine collections at home and again in the hospital. In addition, Cohen and Lazarus' Recovery Index (1973) was used to measure recovery from surgery and was rated at the time of discharge. The results indicated no relationship between defense effectiveness and cortisol production rates in the OPD, and an inverse relationship between cortisol and defense effectiveness under the stress of hospitalization. Effectiveness of coping was also found to be related to adjustment to the ward but not to recovery from surgery. Children who use intellectualization as their major defense were found to cope best with the hospital experience while children who used denial and displacement coped most poorly. Rigidity of defenses was also found to influence effectiveness of coping under stress. Four different groups of children emerged, suggesting four different types of reactions to the hospital experience. Results were discussed with regard to previous studies in the fields of psychosomatic research and hospitalization of children. The relation of psychodynamic theory and child development to issues of hospitalization and surgery was explored. Suggestions for further research were also discussed.

271. Knight, R. B., Atkins, A., Eagle, C. J., Evans, N., Finkelstein, J. W., Fukushima, D., Katz, J., & Weiner, H. Psychological stress, ego defenses, and coritsol production in children hospitalized for elective surgery. Psychosomatic Medicine, 1979, 41(1), 40-49.

This study was designed to investigate the relationship between the effectiveness of coping mechanisms and physiological indicators of distress in children faced with the experience of hospitalization and surgery. Twenty-five children between the ages of seven and eleven were studied in the out-patient department, two weeks before surgery, and again during their hospital stay. Effectiveness of defenses and defense style was measured by a clinical interview and by the Rorschach test. Cortisol production rates were measured by the analysis of 24-hour urine collections at home and again in the hospital. Ward adjustment was also rated by a ward questionnaire. The results indicated no relationship between defense effectiveness and cortisol production rates in the out-patient department and an inverse relationship between cortisol production and defense effectiveness under the stress of hospitalization. Defense style was found to correlate with coping under stress. Four different groups of children emerged, suggesting four different types of reaction to the hospital experience.

272. Komrower, G. The care of children in hospital (letter to the editor). British Medical Journal, 1979, 2(6191), 665.

This letter strongly urges the establishment of more facilities specifically for hospitalized children based on a policy report by Lady Marre's group. The principle so strongly underlined by Lady Marre and her colleagues is that the care of children should be in the hands of people who are deeply concerned with children and, whether they are physicians, surgeons, nurses, technicians, or domestic and portering staff, have elected to work with this age group. Although the comments and recommendations are concerned with cancer in childhood, they are equally applicable to the management of all chronic long-term illnesses and handicaps which are responding to therapy in a way that was thought impossible some years ago.

273. Korsch, B. M. The child and the operating room. Anesthesiology, 1975, 43(2), 251-257.

Pediatricians, parents and others involved in the care of sick children have become increasingly aware that illness, hospitalization, and most especially surgical operations have significant emotional and psychological impact on the growing child. Regression, depression, withdrawal, anxiety, increased dependency, and other behavior problems sometimes occur in children following hospitalization and/or surgery. Family relationships, especially parental relationships with the sick child himself, cultural patterns, and economic background of the family influence strongly the manner in which the young child adapts to the experiences of surgery and hospitalization. The attitude of the caretaking personnel in hospitals also makes for differences in adaptation on the part of the patient and his family. A general outline of growth and development, especially in respect to issues relevant to illness, hospitalization and surgery, needs to be kept in mind by those caring for infants, children, and adolescents in hospital so that the patients' behavior can be considered in context of the developmental stage and responded to in an appropriate manner.

274. Korsch, B. M. Issues in humanizing care for children. American Journal of Public Health, 1978, 68(9), 831-832.

This editorial discusses the curious paradox that whereas new research findings of a biologic or technologic nature are incorporated into medical practice promptly--sometimes before being truly tested--research relating to the psychologic welfare of children is applied to the care of children in hospitals and to pediatric practice at a slow rate against much resistance and with many distortions. Some of the barriers that exist to increased parental involvement in the care of the hospitalized child are noted, and suggestions for change discussed.

275. Koss, T., & Teter, M. Welcoming a family when a child is hospitalized. MCN: American Journal of Maternal Child Nursing, 1980, 5 (1), 51-54.

This article describes the development of an "admission assessment and teaching unit" designed to assess and prepare the child and his family for admission to hospital, which has as its goals the following: (1) to alleviate some stress associated with hospitalization through pre- and post-surgical teaching, explanation of hospital routines and procedures, and orientation of the patient and family to the surroundings; (2) to make an initial physical and emotional assessment of the child for the purpose of acting immediately on secondary problems; (3) to encourage the family to participate in the child's care; (4) to communicate pertinent information to the nursing staff so that they are immediately familiar with the family and its problems; and (5) to lighten the workload on nursing staff by completing routine admission procedures and, with parents, write an initial plan of care.

276. Kueffner, M. Passage through hospitalization of severely burned, isolated school-age children. Communicating Nursing Research, 1975, 7, 181-197.

This study investigated how staff and parents can best function in relation to young hospitalized burn victims. The data indicate that parents are able to function in difficult and trying situations and can assist in the needs of the child. For the researcher, and for the reader, this study affords a graphic and dramatic picture of the experience of severely burned, isolated children and their families during initial hospitalization after a truly catastrophic occurrence.

277. Kueffner, M. C. A qualitative study of the passage through hospitalization of severely burned, isolated school-age children (Doctoral dissertation, University of California, San Francisco, 1973). Dissertation Abstracts International, 1975, 35(9-B), 4520.

This is an exploratory study of the behavior of six severely burned, isolated school-age children during initial hospitalization. Subjects were 5.8 to 9.5 years of age with second and third degree burns varying in extent from 20% to 75% of body surface area. Two children were isolated alone in a room on a pediatric ward of two separate hospitals. Four children were isolated together on a six-bed ward of a burn unit. Analysis of the data was a continuous process. Three key categories were abstracted which conceptualized the data. Pain was identified as a major factor influencing behavior. Aloneness, integral to the burn experience as well as isolation, was found to be of two types: (1) imposed or engendered by the hospital, and (2) selected or managed by the child. Loss was discovered to be part of the experience of each of the subjects and was subdivided into four classes: (1) possible loss of bodily self by death, (2) loss of parents by separation, (3) loss of control over self and the environment, and (4) loss of attractiveness. Three stages were designated as occurring between the accident and the time of discharge from the hospital. Stage 1 (Agony) begins with the hospitalization and ends when the child senses he is improving and will survive. Stage II (Hope) begins when the child senses that he is improving and will survive and ends when a fairly definite time for discharge has been designated. Stage III (Reorganization) begins when a date for discharge is set and ends when the child leaves the hospital for home.

278. Kum, E., & Ilgen, N. Hospitalization of the child. Part I. Turkish Journal of Pediatrics, 1977, 19(1-2), 1-15.

It is not only the separation from his mother and family, or the impatience of the child that affects him when hospitalized. The quite unfamiliar place, the hospital, is also a source which affects him emotionally. Such environmental change means for the infant changes in sensory and social stimulations. In addition, hospitalization means becoming subject to unpredictable, frightening, and painful experiences. Some of the factors which relate to the way the child handles stress, anxiety and tension provoked by the hospitalization, as discussed in this article, include: (1) The nature of the illness, its acuteness, severity and duration; (2) The type of symptoms, the degree of discomfort involved in diagnostic procedures; (3) The parents' attitudes about the cause of separation; (4) Interaction of individual potentials, as the hereditary factors and the mechanisms for adjusting to new environment; (5) Age of the child or the stage of development at the time of illness or hospitalization and their effect on the reactions; (6) The quality of care he receives in the hospital and the child's relations with nurses and physicians; (7) His previous experiences; and (8) His fear and fantasies of the surgery and the anesthesia.

279. Kum, E., & Ilgen, N. Hospitalization of the child. Part II. Turkish Journal of Pediatrics, 19(3-4), 109-117.

Hospitalization requires extra tasks from the child when his capacity already is handicapped by his illness and separation from his familiar surroundings. The negative impacts of these factors on both parents and children receive proper attention in most hospitals of the western countries. Certain changes in regular hospital practices seem to minimize the adverse effects of hospitalization and separation of children. Some of these policies and procedures as discussed in this article include: (1) If possible, the mother should stay with and care for her child; (2) If the mother cannot stay with and take care of the child, the child should receive the frequent care and attention of a limited number of hospital personnel; (3) Lengthen the visiting hours and shorten the stays in hospital; (4) Hospital experience must be modified to meet the child's endurance; and (5) Preparation of the child for hospital admission and treatment is crucial.

280. Kunzman, L. Some factors influencing a young child's mastery hospitalization. Nursing Clinics of North America, 1972, 7(1), 13-26.

There are significant areas of difference between the child and the adult in respect to the experience of hospitalization. Comprehending the impact of hospitalization on the child requres a better understanding of how he interprets his experience. It requires a comparison of the child's situation at home with his situation when hospitalized. Separation for the young child intensifies the traumatic effects of the hospital experience. Encouragement of rooming-in for parents seems clearly indicated from the point of view of the child, parent, and preventive health care. Helping the child toward mastery of his experience is a valuable asset for his growth and development. Play can be utilized as a resource to help the child cope with his experience. It provides an opportunity to deal with his feelings that he cannot express in words, provides some physical activity, and offers the opportunity for learning and growth.

281. Lampe, J. Parental visiting of sick infants: The effect of living at home prior to hospitalization. Pediatrics, 1977, 59(2), 294-296.

The frequency of parental visiting was studied to determine the effects of a short period of care at home and the presence of a visible congenital anomaly on parent-to-infant attachment. The underlying assumption for the first factor is that bonding develops most readily in the intimacy of the home, where the parent has privacy, continuous contact, and full responsibility for care-taking. A visible malformation, on the other hand, would be expected to interfere with the development of attachment. The study was conducted on a 30-bed infant unit during two two-week periods, one month apart. The parental visiting rate was determined for all 44 children present on the unit during these two periods for at least six days. The analysis of the visiting rates was based on the combined data from both two-week studies. There was a statistically significant difference in visiting rates between the parents of children who had been home for two or more weeks prior to hospitalization and those whose children had not. Although parents visited an infant with a visible congenital anomaly somewhat less than parents visited a baby with no malformation or with a nonvisible congenital defect (for example, congenital cardiac or renal abnormalities), the difference was not significant.

282. Landsman, E. The function of a play program in pediatrics. Pediatric Annals, 1972, 1(3), 64-69.

Illness and hospitalization, usually accompanied by separation from the parent as well, are a traumatic interruption in a child's life and as such present a situation of particular challenge to the many professionals involved in the care of the child in the hospital. The strange and frightening procedures of the medical institution not only painfully interrupt the normal life of the child, but usually hospitalization deprives him of the opportunity to cope with stressful situations in ways that are age appropriate. This article discusses the role of play in the hospitalized child's life. Play in the hospital is of particular importance during a time of stress, and enables the child to continue with as many aspects of normal, healthy growth as his medical situation permits.

283. Leff, P. T., & Chan, J. M. Reflections of a medical student in a Child Life Program. Journal of the Association for the Care of Children in Hospitals, 1977, 5(3), 20-24.

This article describes a Child Life Program at State University Hospital, Downstate Medical Center in New York, which was set up as a seven-day-a-week program. Objectives were twofold: (1) to meet the developmental, emotional and intellectual needs of hospitalized children; and (2) to meet the educational needs of students interested in child health care. Opportunities are provided in the program for observation and practice while the students are learning theoretical concepts in child health, child study, and developmental psychology. The case of a six-year-old boy disfigured by scars is discussed.

284. Lehberger, L. Responses of an adolescent to immobilization during hospitalization. Maternal-Child Nursing Journal, 1973, 2(3), 189-195.

This report discusses the emotional difficulties and accomplishments of a 15-year-old male after 18 months of immobilization. As a result of this experience feelings of helplessness, deprivation, and depression aggravated the identity and independence crises typically felt by a normal adolescent.

285. Lehman, E. J. The effects of rooming-in and anxiety on the behavior of preschool children during hospitalization and follow-up (Doctoral dissertation, Cornell University, 1975). Dissertation Abstracts International, 1975, 36(6-B), 3052.

This study was concerned with the reactions of children who were hospitalized for tonsillectomy and/or adenoidectomy. Specifically, the effect of having mothers room-in and the child's anxiety-proneness were examined in relation to aggression, post-operative complications, and the child's behavior two weeks after his hospital stay. Subjects were 48 children ranging in age from three to five years, who were from intact families, and had no previous hospitalizations. There were 12 subjects in each of four categories: rooming-in and non-rooming-in boys, with the same division for girls. One finding of this study is that rooming-in children are more aggressive in the hospital, both to their mothers and to the nurses. It was also hypothesized that at follow-up the rooming-in child would show fewer behavioral disturbances than his non-rooming-in counterpart. There was a trend in this direction, again suggesting the importance of the mother's presence in terms of the child's behavior. It was also hypothesized that the high-anxiety-prone child would be less aggressive in the hospital, have more post-operative complications, more negative post-hospital behavioral changes, and more aggressive post-hospitalization behavior than would a child with a lower anxiety level. These hypotheses were not borne out. It was also hypothesized that separation from the child's mother would augment the effects of the child's anxiety proneness. Only the post-operative complications suggested an interaction of anxiety with rooming-in.

286. Leonhard, K. Can childhood schizophrenia develop out of hospitalization? Psychiatrica Clinica, 1978, 11(3), 170-179.

Out of 59 childhood schizophrenics examined, 11 had fallen ill as early as within the first years of their lives. Seven of these had been confined to a hospital or a similar institution when the illness set in. Two other children were congenitally blind or deaf and, owing to this fact, were largely deprived of communication with their environment. It was possible to diagnose schizophrenia even though the patients were mentally retarded. It seems that lack of communication within the first years of life can not only produce mental retardation but also provoke childhood schizophrenia.

287. Lerner, M. J., Haley, J. V., Hall, D. S., & McVarish, D. Hospital care-by-parent: An evaluative look. Medical Care, 1972, 10(5), 430-436.

The findings of an evaluative study of an experimental pediatric unit in which routine nursing care is accomplished by parents are summarized. The study focused on communication between parent and physician, effects of hospitalization on the patient and his family, and the impact of the unit on medical students. In general, both parents and physicians were satisfied with the communications but "errors" were uncovered, especially in regard to the child's diagnosis, prognosis, and after-care. Also, parents were pleased with their other experiences on the unit and with the opportunity it provided for them to stay with their children. Disruptions of family life were minimal. Most medical students expressed approval of the unit as a care facility and preferred it to the more traditional pediatric ward as a teaching experience.

288. Levine, M. I. A pediatrician's view. Pediatric Annals, 1972, 1(3), 6-9.

A pediatrician discusses the differences between hospital care and parental visiting policies of the 1940's and the advances that have recently come as a result of the gradual understanding of the emotional needs of children in hospital. The hospital of today should no longer be for the child an experience of terror, anxiety, fear or even dreariness and rejection. With doctors and nurses alike understanding the needs of children at different developmental levels and also recognizing the needs of their parents, the hospital experience can even be in most respects rewarding and pleasurable as well as beneficial.

289. Levitin, N. Brightening children's hospital stay: RT plus paint! Hospital Progress, 1977, 58(9), 115-116.

This article describes a recreational therapy program on the pediatric unit at Timken Mercy Hospital in Canton, Ohio. The woman who operates as the hospital's recreational therapist feels strongly that art and recreational therapy are closely related. The hospital reports improved patient morale and employee appreciation as benefits of the wall art decoration which was used to transform the pediatric unit into a cheerful and colorful area.

290. Levy, M. D. Psychological factors affecting the treatment and hospitalization of chronically ill children (Doctoral dissertation, California School of Professional Psychology, 1975). Dissertation Abstracts International, 1976, 36(11-B), 5802.

The objective of this study was to evaluate the efficacy of three independent variables, locus of control, cognitive style, and chronic illness, as possible predictors of the child's response to treatment and hospitalization. Seventy-six children, male and female, between the ages of four through eleven years, all currently hospitalized with diagnoses of chronically fatal or chronically non-fatal participated. Five major hypotheses, including a total of 15 predictions, were generated in an attempt to measure the hospitalized child's mood level, self-esteem, anxiety and alienation as a function of his fatal-nonfatal status, locus of control and cognitive style. Analysis of variance included both between and within group comparisons. Independent variables utilized the Oltman (1954) Portable Rod-and-Frame as a measure of cognitive style, and the Children's Health Control Scale as a measure of the child's locus of control. Dependent instruments included a hospital mood index, a self-esteem measure utilizing a technique developed by Zelen (1968) as a measure of the child's reported self-worth. Measures of anxiety and alienation included the use of a 3-D Doll House technique developed and extensively reported by Spinetta (1972). The data from the study warranted several important conclusions: (1) That locus of control and cognitive style may meaningfully predict a chronically ill child's attempt to cope with his illness and hospitalization, and (2) The manner in which a child with a particular locus of control or cognitive style attempts to cope is often dependent upon whether or not a chronically ill child has a fatal or nonfatal prognosis.

291. Lewis, B. E. The who, what, why, when, where, and how of effecting environmental change in pediatric medical settings. Journal of the Association for the Care of Children in Hospitals, 1978, 6(3), 4-10.

Professionals who work with children and their families in medical settings commonly find that the surroundings are uncomfortably institutional or so depressing that work and medical care are actually impeded. Once aware of a nonsupportive environment, professionals often experience confusion as to where to begin to make changes in it. The author, an environmental planner, discusses major concerns that center around the following questions: First, what do professionals need to know about the environment in order to make changes? Second, how can space be changed and redesigned with a minimum of effort and expense? Third, when should the advice of a professional be sought, what kind of designer should be consulted, and how is the talent of such a person (or group) best utilized?

292. Lewis, N. I probably won't have all the luxuries in the world. Journal of the Association for the Care of Children in Hospitals, 1978, 7(1), 28-32.

The author discusses and illustrates the use of art and creative writing by hospitalized children. These activities give them an opportunity to constructively express emotions and conflicts engendered by the experience of illness and hospitalization. Examples of the usefulness of this therapeutic technique are presented and discussed.

293. Lincoln, L. Effects of illness and hospital procedures on body image in adolescents: A review of the literature. Maternal-Child Nursing Journal, 1978, 7(2), 55-60.

Literature reviewed for this paper pertains to selected aspects of body image, such as personal space and body boundary, and effects of illness and hospital procedure on body-image during adolescence.

294. Lindheim, R., Glaser, H. H., & Coffin, C. Changing hospital environments for children. Cambridge, Massachusetts: Harvard University Press, 1972.

Many children, particularly younger ones, experience ill effects from being hospitalized. The syndrome called institutionalism can smother the distinctive style and individual pattern of growth of almost any child. This book attempts to develop design guidelines that can be of help in generating environments sympathetic to the needs of children of different ages who are required to live away from home for medical reasons. Alternatives to hospitalization are first explored. Where these are lacking, ways to bridge the gap between the community and the hospital are identified. The specific developmental needs of infants, toddlers and preschoolers, school-age children, and adolescents are then discussed in relation to their environmental needs, and on this basis design guidelines for hospitals are drawn up. The needs of parents and staff in the hospital environment are also examined, with particular emphasis placed on nursing unit design.

295. Lindquist, I. Therapy through play. London: Arlington Books, 1977.

In the definition of the author, "play therapy," often used in the book, is "the pedagogical and psychological care of children and parents during their stay in the hospital." The book's chapters deal separately with equipment used for various ages and impairments, and with the great variety of different approaches to children with practically all types of dysfunction of illness. The book does not bring any particular psychological theories from which to embark. It is based on the intuititve understanding and individual needs of patients and on the author's art to get through the defenses of children. Through this approach the hospital stay can become a time for growth. One suggestion may be especially helpful for hospital workers: the "lending library" of equipment and books for handicapped children upon their return home. The importance of the interaction of the whole team is brought out in this volume, especially the support the medical director of pediatrics can give a beginning program. Three forewords stress this point.

296. Lindquist, I. Influencing attitudes toward children's emotional care. Journal of the Association for the Care of Children in Hospitals, 1981, 9(3), 73-76.

This article examines the use of play therapy to stimulate hospitalized children by linking up their thoughts to a normal, healthy life instead of dealing exclusively with disease.

297. Linn, S. Puppets and hospitalized children: Talking about feelings. Journal of the Association for the Care of Children in Hospitals, 1977, 5(4), 5-11.

Puppetry is established in many hospitals as a technique for preparing children individually and in groups for specific hospital procedures. It has broader possibilities as a creative tool for open-ended dialogues with children about feelings evoked by hospitalization, separation, loss of control, operations, etc. Because puppets are so useful, helping children identify, clarify, and verbalize their feelings, and because the author does not believe that one has to be a professional puppeteer to work with puppets in this manner, this article discusses different ways in which she has successfully used puppets as tools for talking with hospitalized children.

298. Linn, S. Puppet therapy in hospitals: Helping children cope. Journal of the American Medical Women's Association, 1978, 33(2), 61-65.

Hospitalization is frightening and confusing for children. While children vary in their ability to cope successfully with hospitalization, all of them need adult intervention to help them positively assimilate the experience. This article describes a program which uses puppet therapy to help children prepare for surgery and catheterization, and helps them deal with their feelings and concerns afterward. A child engaged in spontaneous but supervised puppet play with a sensitive adult has an active verbal release for frustration and tensions. At the same time he can explore frightening thoughts and feelings and gain mastery over a confusing and overwhelming environment. Puppetry is a therapeutic tool particularly suited to helping hospitalized children cope with invasive and/or painful procedures, loss of autonomy, and separation from home. Because puppets are a means of eliciting meaningful material quickly they are especially well suited to hospitals where the length of stay may be quite short.

299. Liviskie, S. Definition of body boundaries after burn injury. Maternal-Child Nursing Journal, 1973, 2(2), 101-109.

Burn injury and the ensuing treatment procedures can foster disruption of body boundary concept by altering the appearance, sensation and perception of the body surface. Submersion in the whirlpool bath and removal of dressings produced a sense of loss of boundaries in themselves and in the pain sensations these procedures produced. When there is pain on the body surface, the body image becomes distorted at the point of pain; there is a sensation of swelling. The painful area of the body is pushed out of the body image. Also, defects may be eliminated by disowning the affected body part. The ability to disown one's body parts presents a threat to the body integrity; and there exists a general fear of dismemberment. This article presents a case study of one hospitalized three-year-old boy treated for burn injuries. He disowned his defective, painful body surface, and, therefore, experienced further loss of body boundaries and senations of disintegration.

300. Lockwood, N. L. The effect of situational doll play upon the preoperative stress reactions of hospitalized children. ANA Clinical Sessions, Miami. New York: Appleton-Century-Cofts, 1970, 113-120.

The purpose of the study reported here was to ascertain if situational doll play between the child and the nurse would alter the level of stress and anxiety which the child experiences during the period of hospitalization prior to surgery. The population selected for this study consisted of 20 children aged four to six years who were admitted to the pediatric ward for elective surgery during a selected four-week period. The Hospital Picture Test, a thematic apperception test involving eight cards, was used to determine the level of fantasy stress reactions and the focus of stress reactions. It was concluded that situational doll play as employed in this study did not affect the preoperative level of stress experienced by children participating in this study. While the total stress scores were not changed, the anxiety-defense of children treated with situational doll play decreased significantly, and the focus of the stress reaction significantly increased in the doctors and/or medical procedures category. The author reports the following implications based on this study: (1) The pediatric nurse should expand her knowledge and increase her skills in the use of situational doll play; (2) The pediatric nurse should seek to identify the coping mechanisms of children six years of age and older and give each child support in his efforts to master the situation in his own way; and (3) The pediatric nurse might well expand the scope of her practice to include observing and serving the child in his own home prior to admission to the hospital for surgery.

301. Loomis, W. G. Management of children's emotional reactions to severe body damage (burns). Clinical Pediatrics, 1970, 9(6), 362-367.

Severely burned children experience profound emotional as well as physical trauma, and the management of the latter seems well worthy of study. Accordingly, the author saw professionally every burned child who was hospitalized at Colorado General Hospital for more than one day during nearly two years. This report discusses 16 such patients of whom eight, all under five years old, were followed for a prolonged time.

302. Lord, R., & Schowalter, J. Visiting on an adolescent ward. Journal of the Association for the Care of Children in Hospitals, 1979, 8(1), 5-9.

This report discusses the psychological implications of parents', siblings', and friends' patterns of visiting hospitalized children, based upon an interview-format survey of the attitudes of 200 hospitalized children aged 11-16 and 100 parents of hospitalized children.

303. Lowenstein, H. The handling of distress. Nursing Times, 1972, 68(43), 1363-1364.

The author of this article, who has worked on a study of the reaction of small children admitted to hospital, reports on a new film project based on the distress cry of the small child. In this article he takes a look at the nurse-mother-child interrelationship and finds three ways of tackling distress.

304. Lowery, C. H. Preparing children for the hospital. American Family Physician, 1975, 12(3), 136-137.

This article discusses preparation of children for a stay in the hospital. Preparation for this drastic change in a child's life-style is possible regardless of the size of the hospital, and adequate preparation is urged since it has been shown to produce beneficial effects. The author maintains that the task of preparation cannot be delegated to parents, many of whom are incapable of accomplishing this responsibility, but instead should come in the form of assistance from the physician and other paramedical personnel. Aids which are now available for preparing children for hospitalization and surgery are described.

305. Lowit, I. M. Social and psychological consequences of chronic illness in children. Developmental Medicine and Child Neurology, 1973, 15(1), 75-77.

Chronic disease in childhood affects the psycho-social development of the child in ways which must be recognized by those concerned with him if he is to achieve optimal development. Certain psychological effects are associated with the disease process--evidence of an inherent tendency towards synthesis and integration shaping the personality of the child to fit his capacities and needs. This article suggests that it is useful to regard the diagnosis of chronic illness in a child as a "crisis situation" of a special type which merits the investment of skilled manpower. Such a crisis forces a reorganization of family life, and rigidly maladaptive and defensive modes of coping are temporarily disrupted so that, with therapeutic intervention, healthier and more satisfying family patterns can emerge. The skill to assess the emotional resources of the child and his family and to plan for treatment should be part of the total diagnostic and treatment process.

306. Luciano, K. B. Components of planned family-centered care. Nursing Clinics of North America, 1972, 7(1), 41-52.

Family-centered nursing is a multi-dimensional approach to pediatric care. A systematic nursing process must be utilized to meet the dynamic needs of the hospitalized child and his family. Interventions must be planned on the basis of the family's perceptions about the child's illness and treatment and their ability to cope with this life experience. Nursing care activities need to be family-oriented, individualized, and coordinated. The implementation of family-centered care can offer the pediatric nurse a tremendous feeling of satisfaction by providing feedback and meaning to her goal-directed care.

307. Luciano, K. B. Staff development: Toward the implementation of family-centered care. Nursing Clinics of North America, 1972, 7(1), 75-82.

The most important prerequisite for implementing family-centered care is the preparedness of nurses to function within this system. The educational program must be developed on the basis of behavioral objectives. Teaching content and methods have to satisfy the participants' needs for security and self-esteem during the process of learning new behaviors. The inservice educator must provide a climate in which support and feedback exist for encouraging nurses to realize their potentials for family-centered nursing care. Nursing administrators must give constant support to nurses experiencing changes in their role and adopting new patterns of nursing interventions.

308. Luciano, K. The who, when, where, what and how of preparing children for surgery. Nursing, 1974, 4(11), 64-65.

One of the most satisfying aspects of a pediatric nurse's job is watching a child master his fears and anxieties about a scheduled operation. The nurse truly fulfills the role of a helping person when she assists the child and his family to cope with the potentially traumatic experience of surgery. Preparing a child for surgery must be based on several factors: the age or developmental level of the child, his previous experiences with health professionals and hospitals, the operation to be performed, postoperative care, and the expected length of hospitalization. For the child undergoing a first hospitalization and surgery, the required nursing care to reduce anxiety is compounded. This article presents suggestions and considerations when planning preoperative preparation of children for hospitalization and surgery. Specific recommendations are made and a Surgery Preparation Guide for the day before surgery and the day of surgery is presented.

309. MacCarthy, D. Communication between children and doctors. Developmental Medicine and Child Neurology, 1974, 16(3), 279-285.

The author gives a personal view on communication between pediatricians and child patients, and discusses ways in which this special relationship might be enhanced. Case studies are presented to illustrate principles outlined by the author.

310. Magrab, P. R., & Bronheim, S. The child-life model and pediatric hospitalization. Journal of Pediatric Psychology, 1976, 1(4), 7-8.

In this article a multidisciplinary model is suggested for dealing with the impact of hospitalization on children. The team includes the physician, nurse, psychologist, social worker, child-life specialist, consulting psychiatrist, and ward teacher, who work together towards a positive mental health approach to the hospital experience.

311. Manheim, L. Pillow play with hospitalized children: Three case studies. Journal of the Association for the Care of Children in Hospitals, 1980, 9(2), 41-45.

This article describes the work of a student intern who worked with handicapped children for three months at Shriners Hospital in San Francisco. The children at Shriners range in age from two to 15 years and display various orthopedic disorders. Average length of stay in the hospital is approximately 20 days. The paper draws upon journal entries and examines the effects of play sessions on three individual children.

312. Marino, B. L. When nurses compete with parents. Journal of the Association for the Care of Children in Hospitals, 1980, 8(4), 94-98.

The problem of nurses and parents competing for the baby is subtle and potentially damaging to the family. Protective feelings can distort the intentions of parents who are caught in their own feelings of inadequacy and ambivalence. By opening communication, and reinforcing the parents' skills the two groups can pool their resources for the ultimate benefit of the family. The author discusses three approaches nurses can take to prevent competition with parents: (1) help bolster the attachment process between parent and child; (2) deal with the ambivalent feelings that foster a competitive atmosphere; and (3) provide parents with opportunities to learn how to care for their children.

313. Mason, E. A. Hospital and family cooperating to reduce psychological trauma. Community Mental Health Journal, 1978, 14(2), 153-159.

This article discusses some of the advantages in increasing parent involvement during hospitalization and in techniques such as one-day surgery for reducing the length of hospital stays and the potential for psychological trauma. Not only should these programs be encouraged, but this flexibility should be extended to the x-ray unit and even the recovery room, where parent involvement is equally appropriate. Many hospital practices can be demystified and demythologized. This is demonstrated in the film, "We Won't Leave You," discussed in this article. The film was made of one child's experience with outpatient herniorraphy after being held by her mother during induction of anesthesia. The film documents one hospital's effort to meet the psychological needs of parents and children; it also helped change inpatient procedures.

314. Mattson, A. Long-term physical illness in childhood: A challenge to psychosocial adaptation. *Pediatrics*, 1972, *50*(5), 801-811.

This paper reviews long-term disorders in childhood from the standpoint of the attendant psychologic stresses and the related adaptational techniques used by the child and his parents in their attempt to master their negative and distressing emotions. Such techniques include the use of cognitive functions, motor activity, emotional expression, and certain psychologic defenses. Clinical examples illustrate how these coping mechanisms can support or hinder good psychosocial adaptation due to the degree of their employment and the nature of the parent-child relationship. Children with chronic illness as well as their parents show a rather predictable sequential pattern in adapting to their difficult situation. The parents' early acceptance of their child's disability and its impact on the family is crucial in promoting a healthy personality development of the child.

315. Mattson, A. Psychologic aspects of childhood asthma. *Pediatric Clinics of North America*, 1975, *22*(1), 77-88.

Child psychiatry has a definite but selective role in the management of asthmatic children. Referral for psychosocial evaluation of a family with an asthmatic child is indicated in the following situations: (1) children in whom emotional factors seem to be of precipitating and aggravating importance; (2) children whose asthma perpetuates individual and family psychopathology and maladaptation; (3) behavioral problems in a child seemingly unrelated to his asthma. Psychiatric intervention may be oriented toward prevention of emotionally triggered and aggravated symptoms, modification of the child's and the family's attitudes toward his illness, and alleviation of a concurrent behavior disorder. Frequently, all three directions are pursued. Systematic, long-term evaluations of the effectiveness of various psychologic approaches to the modification of childhood asthma are sorely needed.

316. Mattson, A., & Weisberg, I. Behavioral reactions to minor illness in preschool children. Pediatrics, 1970, 46(4), 604-610.

Over a three-year period 35 preschool children were observed during minor physical illness at home while they were cared for by their mothers. The children came from one pediatrician's private practice and had no history of chronic illness or hospital admission. A total of 76 periods of illness were observed. During the acute phase of illness all children showed some temporary loss of age-appropriate behavior. Particularly striking were the changes in the children's relationship with their mothers. These changes constituted two types of reactions which were related to age. Reaction 1, predominant among the ill two-year-olds, was characterized by the child's clinging, whiny dependence, while children over the age of three tended to show Reaction 2. Its main feature was a self-contained, rather undemanding state. During convalescence all children demonstrated a few days of irritable, impatient behavior. The preschool child's reactions to acute illness at home appear to change with age in an orderly continuum toward self-contained, rather independent behavior. The findings allow for a discussion of the possible role of minor illness in promoting the young child's reality sense and responsibility for the care of his body.

317. McBride, M. M. & Sack, W. H. Emotional management of children with acute respiratory failure in the intensive care unit: A case study. Heart/Lung, 1980, 9(1), 98-102.

The purpose of this article is to describe in some detail various interventions utilized during the hospitalization of a five and a half year old male child with Guillain-Barré syndrome which demonstrate a comprehensive team approach in dealing with emotional issues of young, totally paralyzed children. This case report emphasizes the emotional needs of children during protracted illness and describes in some detail practical nursing interventions that can be carried out in any intensive care setting. The particular interventions of the pediatric/child psychiatric liaison team are described here and related to their conceptual foundations. With a solid understanding of the child's emotional development, it is possible to improvise such methods so that comprehensive nursing care can be achieved in an intensive care setting.

318. McCabe, M. C. Innovations in a pediatric unit. Hospital Progress, 1970, 51, 26.

This article reports on several innovations implemented at St. John's Hospital, Springfield, Missouri. An attractive mural has been added to the pediatric unit as well as new curtains and gaily colored sheets. The personnel on the pediatric unit now wear dresses in pastel shades with a name tag that shows name and position. An effort has been made to help parents by providing a coffee cart where personnel serve anxious parents. Relaxing chairs have been made available to parents who may wish to hold a sick child. The Kraft Kloset is a source of never-ending delight to patients on the unit. The Kloset furnishes material for making simple objects and seasonal displays. In an effort to make children feel at home, the unit has acquired a pair of gerbils, which the children delight in feeding and watching. Another means of keeping children happy is to allow their brothers and sisters to visit them. These innovations have met with marked success. They have helped patients lose their fear of hospitals and to look back at their time at St. John's as an exciting experience.

319. McCue, K., Wagner, M., Hansen, H., & Rigler, D. Survey of a developing health care profession: Hospital "play" programs. Journal of the Association for the Care of Children in Hospitals, 1978, 7(1), 15-22.

The purpose of this investigation was to evaluate the status of child life/recreation therapy programs in pediatric hospitals. The investigation involved obtaining information on: (1) geographic division and titles of programs; (2) general structure of programs; (3) program philosophies; (4) staffing structure, qualifications, and salary; and (5) how the programs are perceived by the institutions. The relationships and interactions among the various items of information gathered were also examined. The one fact clearly established by this report is that there is immense variation in all aspects, both operational and philosophical, of the staff and organizational positions within the institutions. The needs of pediatric patients have been extensively documented, as have the general effects of hospitalization. Other data relevant to the use of play programs in hospitals are also reported.

320. McDonnell, L. Paraverbal therapy in pediatric cases with emotional complications. American Journal of Orthopsychiatry, 1979, 49 (1), 44-52.

Children often respond to hospitalization with severe anxiety and depression, frequently manifested by withdrawal or hyperactive and aggressive or hostile behavior. The use of paraverbal therapy, a specialized therapeutic approach, is described in the short-term treatment of patients exhibiting emotional disturbances secondary to illness or trauma. Paraverbal therapy is a method of observation, diagnosis, and treatment that uses a variety of expressive media to establish both nonverbal and verbal communication. Paraverbal techniques engage the child by the use of various media, and make the session a pleasureful, stimulating, and reciprocal experience between therapist and child. In this framework, the child is helped to maintain or reestablish relative psychic harmony through experiences of success and mastery, through the appropriate discharge of tensions, and through the communication of painful feelings. Meeting the child's needs, so that he will be better able to cope with his hospital experience, is the goal of paraverbal therapy in a pediatric setting.

321. McElnea, L. Where resident parents are welcome. Nursing Times, 1971, 67(43), 1331-1333.

The vast majority of resident parents who come into hospital with their child feel very unsure of their status and their environment. They are worried about their child and about their relationship with the nursing staff. All these fears diminish when they realize they are welcome. This article describes a program at The Hospital for Sick Children in London which allows parents to stay at the hospital and participate in the care of their sick child.

322. McGillicuddy, M. C. A study of the relationship between mothers' rooming-in during their children's hospitalization and changes in selected areas of children's behavior (Doctoral dissertation, New York University, 1976). Dissertation Abstracts International, 1976, 37 (2-B), 700.

This study compared the effects of short term hospitalization (two to 10 days) on the behavior of children 14 through 48 months of age when the mother roomed in with her child and when she did not. In addition, a group of well and nonhospitalized children were used as controls. The instrument used in data collection was the Vernon and Schulman Behavior Questionnaire. The mothers of all 90 subjects (30 in each group) were administered the questionnaire prior to hospitalization or on the day of admission. This was done again one month following discharge from the hospital. The mothers of the nonhospitalized children were seen at comparable intervals. The results showed that children whose mothers room-in with them during hospitalization demonstrate changes in a positive direction in selected areas of behavior. One month following hospitalization revealed significant positive changes in the areas of general anxiety and regression, eating disturbance and apathy-withdrawal from the time of prehospitalization. Among children whose mothers did not room-in there was significant disturbance in the behavioral areas of separation anxiety, anxiety about sleep, aggression to authority and apathy-withdrawal. Total behavioral change was also regressive at one month following discharge from the hospital.

323. McGuire, M., Shepherd, R., & Greco, A. Hospitalized children in confinement. Pediatric Nursing, 1978, 4(6), 31-35.

Ordinarily, a child's daily life offers a variety of opportunities to develop through play. For the average child in the hospital, these experiences are limited, and if the child is further restricted by confinement to his bed or room, these opportunities can be so severely limited that an interruption in the child's development occurs. This article discusses the concept of confinement with respect to a hospital environment and addresses the following issues: (1) the potential effects of confinement on hospitalized children of different ages; (2) the actual effects of confinement on hospitalized children; and (3) what nurses can do to alleviate the problems with confinement.

324. McKeever, D. A., III. Religious ideation in selected hospitalized children (Doctoral dissertation, Southern Baptist Theological Seminary, 1974). Dissertation Abstracts International, 1974, 35(4-A), 2385-2386.

The purpose of this dissertation was to investigate the religious ideation of hospitalized children. The research focused on the ideation from the perspectives of authority, industry versus inferiority, community or brotherhood, and spontaneous/programmed responses. The hospitalized children were 15 preadolescents ranging in age from seven to eleven years. The control sampling was 15 school children from a local elementary school. Religious ideas were obtained through a semi-clinical interview using projective pictures administered by this writer. Criteria for evaluating the data were specified prior to the evaluative process. The results showed that the hypothesis that religious ideation would be reflective of the subjects' current life situations was affirmed in part. It was affirmed because the religious ideas reflected the stage of development of the children. However, it was not reflective of either specific research sample. The writer could not look at the raw data and pick out the hospitalized children's ideas compared with the school children's ideas. A second hypothesis was not confirmed. The data did not suggest that children facing major crises would tend to be more religiously oriented or give more religious interpretations to their situations than children who were not facing a major crisis. A third hypothesis stated that the religious conceptualization would reflect a concrete level of thinking about religion. This was confirmed by the clinical data. It was found that the older children (nine to eleven years) gave more detailed responses than the younger children (seven to eight years). However, the ideas were largely concrete in nature.

325. McMullen, K. A., Salganicoff, M., & Swierczynski, M. A. Team building and its effects on the hospital and home care of tracheotomized children. Journal of the Association for the Care of Children in Hospitals, 1975, 4(2), 9-13.

The three authors of this article present three aspects of the problem of team building. The history of the team building program instituted at St. Christopher's Hospital for Children in the inner-city community of North Philadelphia is described. The role of a psychologist as a consultant and member of the committee is examined, and the effects of the team building process are discussed.

326. McNemar, A. A child's incorporation of changes in body image following ileal loop diversion. Maternal-Child Nursing Journal, 1972, 1(1), 33-38.

Surgery creates an abrupt change in the body structure and causes disruption of the body image. In order to re-establish interpersonal contacts and self-esteem, the child who undergoes surgery must alter his body image to include the surgical changes in his body structure. The subject of this paper was an energetic nine-and-a-half year old girl who was admitted to a large children's hospital for an elective ileal loop diversion. During the hospitalization the child had to adjust to changes in her body image that included an additional incision, a stoma, an ostomy bag, and internal surgical changes which were not visible to her.

327. Meadow, R. Hospital visiting of children. Proceedings of the Royal Society of Medicine, 1972, 65, 341-342.

Despite repeated recommendations by the Department of Health, only a minority of children in hospital today have unrestricted visiting. This article addresses whether unrestricted visiting is necessary, why it has not been more widely implemented, and what are the problems it creates.

328. Meeks, J. E. Dispelling fears of the hospitalized child. Hospital Medicine, 1970, 6, 77-81.

Hospitalization of a child produces fear at both a rational and irrational level in the youngster and his parents. The irrational fears are more likely to be destructive both in the child's medical management and in long-range disruption of personality development and the parent-child relationship. These irrational concerns tend to be related to the age of the child and should be specifically understood and dealt with according to the needs of the specific developmental phase. Detailed preparation of the youngster so that he knows what to expect during his stay in the hospital is an extremely useful way of dispelling fears, especially in older children. During the hospital stay the child should be encouraged to talk openly and freely about his concerns and, if possible, the younger child should be given the opportunity to play out some of his anxiety. Skillful management of this important part of total medical care should be part of the armamentarium of all physicians who deal with children in a hospital setting. Benefits in improving the hospital management of children and in avoiding a negative impact on their future adjustment justify the effort and additional time required on the part of the doctor.

329. Melamed, B. G., & Siegel, L. J. Reduction of anxiety in children facing hospitalization and surgery by use of filmed modeling. Journal of Consulting and Clinical Psychology, 1975, 43(4), 511-521.

Sixty children about to undergo elective surgery for hernias, tonsillectomies, or urinary-genital tract difficulties were shown on hospital admission either a relevant peer modeling film of a child being hospitalized and receiving surgery or an unrelated control film. Both groups received extensive preparation by the hospital staff. State measures of anxiety, including self-report, behavioral observation, and Palmar Sweat Index, revealed a significant reduction of preoperative (night before) and postoperative (three to four week postsurgery examination) fear arousal in the experimental as compared to the control film group. The parents reported a significant posthospital increment in the frequency of behavior problems in the children who had not seen the modeling film. Trait measures of anxiety did not reflect the group differences due to the hospital experience.

330. Melamed, B. G., Meyer, R., Gee, C., & Soule, L. The influence of time and type of preparation on children's adjustment to hospitalization. Journal of Pediatric Psychology, 1976, 1(4), 31-37.

This report describes the use of film modeling with 48 four to twelve year old children preparing for hospitalization and elective surgery. The successful reduction of the subjects' anxiety held true even in the absence of a large scale preoperative preparation program in the hospital. Older subjects appeared to benefit from seeing the film one week in advance of actual hospitalization. Younger subjects needed more immediate preparation. The effectiveness of the film in reducing anxiety was enhanced when the child observer was similar in age, sex, and race to the child narrator of the film.

331. Meng, A. L. Parents' and children's reactions toward impending hospitalization for surgery. Maternal-Child Nursing Journal, 1980, 9 (2), 83-98.

The purpose of this paper is to report findings from interview data which were obtained as part of a study designed to measure the effect of a preadmission program on children's hospital-related anxiety. The findings reported here relate to parents' assessments of their children's reactions to impending hospitalization and parents' perception of children's needs in relation to psychological preparation for surgery. A total of 59 children and their parents were randomly assigned to the preparation group. Control groups were also employed. The results indicated that parents who have had little or no past experience with hospitalization are poorly equipped to prepare their children for impending hospitalization. Parents in this study perceived their own anxiety as being a greater stress factor than the child's anxiety. The responsibility for psychologically preparing children for hospitalization should be a shared responsibility between parents and health professionals.

332. Menke, E. M. Factors related to children's perception of stress in the hospital (Doctoral disseration, Ohio State University, 1972). Dissertation Abstracts International, 1973, 33(8-A), 4093.

The purpose of this study was to identify the stimuli that children perceive as stressful in the hospital. Concomitantly, the relationship between certain variables and the stimuli that children perceive as stressful in the hospital was studied. In this sample, there was a relationship between the stimuli that the children perceived as stressful and the length of time the children were in the hospital. Likewise, there was a relationship between the stimuli that the children perceived as stressful and their preparation for hospitalization. Additionally, there was a relationship between the stimuli that the children perceived as stressful in the hospital and the following group of variables: children's age, sex, diagnosis, preparation for hospitalization, experience with separation, and the length of hospitalization.

333. Menke, E. M. School-aged children's perception of stress in the hospital. Journal of the Association for the Care of Children in Hospitals, 1981, 9(3), 80-86.

The purpose of this investigation was to study school-aged children's perception of stress as a function of their preparation for hospitalization and the length of their hospitalization. The sample consisted of 50 children (aged six to twelve) who were hospitalized in a children's hospital. The finding of 42 different stresses identified by the sample lends support to the concept that the hospital is a stressful environment for children. The results of this study did not support the hypothesis that there is a relationship between the stimuli children perceive as stressful in the hospital and their preparation for hospitalization. The results of the study did not support statistically the hypothesis that there is a relationship between the stimuli children perceive as stressful in the hospital and the length of time they are hospitalized.

334. Merrington, D. A. The young child in hospital: A health hazard. Australian Family Physician, 1979, 8(12), 1239-1242.

In this paper the author describes a young child most at risk from institutional care, and calls for a new awareness of the emotional needs of young children. The author calls for changes in training programs, for changes in hospital policies, and for a deeper involvement of the mother in the health team when the patient is a young child. The glaring inconsistency now so prevalent in the management of children must be countered by clear positive guidelines and by "unifying principles" which are embodied in legislation. A healthier adult population will then emerge.

335. Millar, T. P. The hospital and the preschool child. Children, 1970, 17, 171-176.

This article considers how psychological disturbances resulting from children's hospitalization can be prevented, or, if that is not possible, how they can be dealt with in the post-hospital period so as to minimize their effect on the psychological health of the child. Two approaches are necessary to prevent or minimize the psychological hazards of hospitalization for young children: (1) to avoid hospitalizing children whenever possible; and (2) to redesign hospital child care practices to reduce the stress of the child's hospital stay as much as possible. The role of the physician in supporting the child and family when the child is discharged and returns home is discussed.

336. Milosavljević, L. J., Kondić-Petrović, K., & Pjanović, Z. Pre- and post-operative anxiety in children. In A. L. Annell (Ed.), Depressive states in childhood and adolescence. New York: Halsted Press, 1972, 207-211.

The aim of the present investigation, prompted by three cases of phobia in tonsillectomized children, was to examine the way children experience this surgical event, to identify the factors operative in the development of psychic disturbances. It was hypothesized that children that were adequately prepared would withstand the operation itself and hospitalization, i.e., separation from their families, more easily. The investigation covered a group of 50 children (28 boys and 22 girls) hospitalized and tonsillectomized in the ORL department of the Institute for Mother and Child Health Protection of Serbia. Their age ranged from three to ten years. The parents of each child were interviewed and among other things information was obtained on how the child had been prepared for the operation, whether this was the first separation from the family and the first stay in hospital. Each child was interviewed before the operation and asked to draw his family and then whatever he wished. On the second or third post-operative day the same procedure was repeated. The parents were interviewed by a paedopsychiatrist, and the children interviewed and their drawings interpreted jointly by the paedopsychiatrist and psychologist. The drawings were used as projective materials to analyse the emotional state of the child at admission, his position in the family and the emotional satisfaction it furnished him. The results (as a whole) showed that with children that were more adequately prepared there were smaller fluctuations in behavior, i.e., in emotional reactions, pre- and post-operatively than with those inadequately prepared or unprepared.

337. Mitchell, E., & Anderson, R. T. Danish child life specialists organize for common concerns. Journal of the Association for the Care of Children in Hospitals, 1978, 7(3), 20-24.

This article compares some of the problems encountered by Danish and American child life specialists: criteria for professional training, continuing education, program development, integration and participation with the medical staff, and increased authority over budgets and decision making. While Danish hospitals exhibit more consistent support and better staffing for child life programs than is commonly found in American hospitals, the recognition of the child life specialist as a professional appears to be better developed in North America. Professional status cannot be attained without specialized training and competent performance. In both Denmark and America, child life specialists are seeking ways to strengthen their work with children in hospitals. The shared experience of both groups could be mutually beneficial.

338. Murphy, D. C. The therapeutic value of children's literature. Nursing Forum, 1972, 11(2), 141-156.

This article discusses the use of bibliotherapy for hospitalized children. The author reports that books can serve a number of nursing care needs of the child including: (1) a means of establishing rapport between the nurse and child; (2) use of books as a tool for growth; (3) the presence of books in the hospital, clinic, or physician's office serves as a source of familiarity, security, and friendliness; (4) books represent a source of credibility for the child; (5) where physical activity is curtailed, listlessness and withdrawal may be offset by a stimulating book; (6) books may assist recovery of the child; and (7) books can offer ideas to help children with other problems superimposed on and further aggravated by illness or hospitalization.

339. Nagai, S. Children in hospitals; two special problems. Dimensions in Health Service, 1979, 56(6), 30, 32.

The care of children with cancer and doctor-parent communication were two topics discussed at a meeting held by the British Columbia affiliate of the Association for the Care of Children in Hospitals at the Vancouver Children's Hospital. This article reviews discussion on these special problems.

340. Nagera, H. Children's reactions to hospitalization and illness. Child Psychiatry and Human Development, 1978, 9(1), 3-19.

This paper describes children's reactions to illness and hospitalizations from a developmental point of view. Taking the latter into account, it becomes easier to understand not only the child's reaction at different ages and the reasons for it, but the nature of the potential damage, that is, where and why it takes place, as well as the resources available to the child that may help, if wisely used, to minimize the potential trauma.

341. Narwold, S. J. Coping with hospitalization through play. Journal of Physical Education and Recreation, 1975, 46(5), 35.

Play is an important part of a child's world enabling communication with others, exploration of the environment, and expression of feelings. When a child is removed from a normal environment and placed in a stressful situation such as a hospital, it is vitally imporrant to keep this link with normal daily routine. A program of recreation therapy should meet the child's needs by providing opportunity to engage in either free play or some sort of directive play. This article describes a program of recreation therapy at the Alfred I. duPont Institute in Wilmington, Delaware, which is aimed at helping children adjust emotionally to the hospital situation, reduce anxiety about procedures performed during hospitalization, come to terms with their physical handicaps, and accept themselves as worthwhile individuals. The methods used in dealing with children vary with age, from nondirective free play for toddlers to specific craft projects for adolescents. Spontaneity and a warm, trusting, nonthreatening atmosphere are stressed.

342. Neff, J. A. Recapitulation of the separation-individuation process in a toddler during hospitalization and home care. Maternal-Child Nursing Journal, 1974, 3(2), 87-102.

The author of this report reviews separation-individuation as a normal phase of development during the first two years of life; the two aspects are complementary and interdependent. The recapitulation of the process in a 21-month-old boy, hospitalized twice for correction of congenital dislocation of the right hip, is described. The boy appeared to work through the various stages of separation-individuation during each of his hospitalizations, with the manifestations shorter and less intense after the second surgery.

343. Nelson, B. S. Ann's postoperative play. Maternal-Child Nursing Journal, 1972, 1(2), 193-196.

This article describes the case of a child three years of age hospitalized for surgical correction of a ventricular septal defect. She held a pacifier in her mouth constantly except when she ate, and her speech was characterized by a high-pitched whine. The child removed the pacifier and spoke in a normal voice tone during play sessions in which she was given a suitcase filled with small toys, dolls representative of family, doctor and nurse, and clinical equipment such as stethoscope, candy pills, etc. Two play interviews are presented to illustrate the child's struggle for mastery of her hospitalization and treatments.

344. Noble, E. Why play? Nursing Times, 1974, 70(15), 534-536.

Play is a natural part of a child's life, a means of developing emotionally, socially and intellectually. In ideal circumstances this development progresses in an orderly and organized manner, each stage of learning and control growing out of the previous one. Giving a child opportunities to play in hospital in a full and meaningful way not only ensures this continuity of development, but also helps to bring a feeling of normality to this strange and often frightening environment. In the pleasurable activity of satisfying play, children in hospital can relax and work out many of their difficulties. As they dramatize their problems and thus come to terms with them, they are able to express their feelings of fear, aggression and despair. This article describes the value of play for hospitalized children, and discusses practical ways of implementing play opportunties in hospital.

345. Noble, E. Hospital schools and parents. Special Education: Forward Trends, 1976, 3(2), 13-15.

This article discusses the involvement of parents in their children's education while in hospital. It can correctly be said that children are normally without their parents during school time, but it must be accepted that having a child in hospital imposes abnormal stress on family life. Suggestions for changes in visiting policy so that parents can be available during their child's school day are made, and the advantages of parent participation are described.

346. Norbeta, S. Caring for children with the help of puppets. MCN: American Journal of Maternal Child Nursing, 1976, 1(1), 22, 23, 26.

Many children are poor patients simply because they have not been prepared for their hospital stay or surgery, and puppets can make their preparation fun. The puppets know everyone in the hospital and they can tell the children all about who works there, what they do, and what it will be like to be a patient. By discussing medical experiences with the puppet, children can talk with someone they see as a peer. This article discusses a puppet program at a residential care center where patients range from two to 14 years of age.

347. O'Donnell, R. L. The psychological effects of childhood on hospitalization: Implications for pediatric health care delivery (Doctoral dissertation, University of Iowa, 1976). Dissertation Abstracts International, 1978, 38(7-B), 3121-3122.

This dissertation presents an analysis of the psychological effects of childhood hospitalization, utilizing data yielded by the implementation of a psychometric test method. The Missouri Children's Picture Series (MCPS) was administered to thirty child hospital patients, ranging in age from five to eleven years, upon admission and again 48 hours later. Additional information was obtained from the patient's medical record, a nurse impression report of level of cooperation, and a visitation record. Level of cooperation and the effect of hospitalization, defined by number and direction of profile changes, served as the behavioral response variables. The patient characteristics and hospital stay variables included: visitation, sex of the child, age, prior hospitalization experience, parental "rejection" and "authoritarian" attitudes (measured by administration of the Parental Attitude Research Instrument), health insurance status, home environment (with whom the child lived), ethnic/racial group, diagnosis, religion, and an MCPS classification of each child's initial testing. Statistically significant relationships were found between: the level of patient cooperation and visitation, and the level of patient cooperation and prior hospitalization experience. In the relationship between prior hospitalization and cooperation, children with some inpatient hospital experience showed significantly higher levels of cooperation than those without such experience. A trend also appeared in the findings of the study indicating an inverse (non-statistically significant) relationship between cooperation and test-defined effect of hospitalization. Children who were less cooperative experienced a less harmful test-defined effect during the test period.

348. Olds, A. R. Psychological considerations in humanizing the physical environment of pediatric outpatient and hospital settings. In E. Gellert (Ed.), Psychosocial aspects of pediatric care. New York: Grune & Stratton, 1978, 111-131.

The physical discomforts of pain, illness, and injury

can be upsetting to anyone. For a child, the anxiety of a visit to the doctor or to the hospital is compounded by the threat of unfamiliar people prepared to impose unknown assaults upon his body, and a frightening institutional setting new to his experience. Experiences in pediatric environments affect three psychological needs of children, parents, and staff: the need to feel comfortable, the need to feel in control of one's self, and the need to be purposefully active. General strategies for the successful design of all types of outpatient and inpatient waiting spaces are examined. The design of playrooms for children is discussed as well.

349. Oremland, E. K., & Oremland, J. D. (Eds.). The effects of hospitalization on children: Models for their care. Springfield, Illinois: Charles C. Thomas, Publisher, 1973.

This book is an interdisciplinary evaluation of the multiple considerations that interrelate in determining the traumatic potential in each experience of hospitalization. Though interdisciplinary, the cornerstone of the discussions is the developmental viewpoint. Though evaluated in multiple contexts, the effects of hospitalization on children presented herewith, are viewed primarily in terms of the specifics of inner experience. The ten chapters represent the contributions of forty-five authors. Topics covered include: (1) trauma vs. experience; (2) separation; (3) cognitive development; (4) regression; (5) specific threats; (6) death; and (7) the family and staff.

350. Ortolani, M. Mothers in residence: Mothers as nursing attendants in a children's hospital in Italy. Clinical Pediatrics, 1970, 9(1), 63-64.

This article describes the advantages of requiring mothers to come into residence when their child is hospitalized. The following points are discussed as benefits to the mother, child, hospital, and community: (1) This prevents anxiety in the child from the hospital experience, and strengthens the mother-child relationship; (2) The mother, always well informed, can give precise information to the doctors and nurses at any time concerning the symptoms and peculiarities of the child, and on the treatments which may have been given in the preceding few hours; (3) The risk of cross-infection is minimized, since each mother generally takes care only of her own child, whereas nurses go from one child to another, and from one room to another; (4) The assistance given by the mothers reduces greatly the number of salaried nurses who must be employed; (5) Recovery and convalescence seem to be speeded up when the mother acts as the nurse; (6) This is a great opportunity for instruction of the mothers in health education; (7) The expenses of the mother staying in the hospital are much less than would be the transportation expenses for daily visits to her sick child; and (8) The mothers acquire confidence in the practical nursing procedures which they have learned at the hospital and teach these to other family members on their return home.

351. Parker, G., & Gibson, C. Development of the hospitalized adolescent anxiety tool. Journal of Pediatric Nursing, 1977, 15(12), 21-24.

The Hospitalized Adolescent Anxiety Tool (HAAT) is a self-appraisal questionnaire for measuring anxiety in the medically hospitalized adolescent. It was designed to be used routinely by the Child Psychiatric Nurse (CPN) at the time of admission for assessment of anxiety in adolescents. The purpose of this article is to discuss the need for the tool and to describe the development and initial pilot testing.

352. Patterson, P. Hospitology: The art and science of rendering hospitalization as benign an experience as possible for a child. Dimensions in Health Service, 1979, 56(5), 12-15.

This article is an attempt to draw material on the hospitalization experience of children together in the form of practical information for both parents and hospital staff on how to render hospitalization as benign and pleasant an experience for children as possible. Topics discussed are: (1) preparation for hospitalization; (2) admission and initial separation; (3) visiting; and (4) post-hospitalization syndrome.

353. Penalver, M. Helping the child handle his aggression. American Journal of Nursing, 1973, 73(9), 1554-1555.

There are many ways a nurse can help to lessen the trauma that hospitalization can give a child. One way is to help him be master of something. For example, the child may be used to some simple ritual which can be carried out easily in the hospital. In addition to giving the child control, the ritual also provides predictability which is directly related to making the child feel secure, and thus reduces his need to express anger or hostility. The nurse can also ask the parents how the child normally reacts to frustrating or challenging situations. This might be helpful in planning for nursing intervention. Case studies are presented to illustrate how these principles can be used to help children deal with their aggression while hospitalized.

354. Perelman, J. An answer to Margaret Heagarty's article, "The pediatric clinic--A challenge." Journal of the Association for the Care of Children in Hospitals, 1975, 4(2), 16-18.

Dr. Heagarty states in her article, "The time has come to begin to apply the principles and ingenuity used to change the mode of care for hospitalized children to the needs of the many children receiving care in our clinics." This article describes a program in effect at the Out-Patient Department at Rainbow Babies' and Children's Hospital, University Hospitals of Cleveland, which has been an innovator in many of its inpatient programs. The Child Life Department is now concentrating on making the Out-Patient Clinic Playroom an exemplary one by combining a secure and relaxing atmosphere with professional psychological support to help meet the in-depth needs of both patients and their families.

355. Peters, B. M. Concepts of hospitalized children about causality of illness and intent of treatment (Doctoral dissertation, University of Pittsburgh, 1975). Dissertation Abstracts International, 1976, 36 (12-B), 6074.

The focus of this study was hospitalized children's concepts of the cause of illness and perceptions of the intent behind treatment. The sample consisted of 24 hospitalized children, eight through ten years of age. The 12 boys and 12 girls were distributed equally among three age groups of eight, nine, and ten years, four of each sex in each age group. Primary sources of data consisted of a projective interview and an interview in which direct questions about his illness were asked of each child. The findings suggested that children of early school-age frequently see people, themselves or others, as causal agents for illness. Girls may tend to internalize, while boys tend to externalize responsibility for illness. Illness and the treatment of illness may be perceived as punishment for the child's behavior. This point of view may be more prevalent in the younger children whose cognition is heavily influenced by precausal structures. There was a greater tendency for the younger children than for the older children to mention self as causing the illness and also to see the intent of treatment as punitive. This trend is compatible with movement toward adult forms of causal concepts and moral judgment as cognitive development progresses.

356. Peters, B. M. Threat appraisal by an adolescent girl undergoing surgical correction of scoliosis. Maternal-Child Nursing Journal, 1976, 5(3), 167-178.

The author analyzed one form of threat appraisal--information seeking questions concerned with hospitalization and treatment procedures--as utilized by a 14 year old female whose medical history (idiopathic scoliosis) seemed to contribute to a high degree of concern about and expectation of complications throughout her treatment. Data analyzed were direct questions asked in the presence of the investigator, who provided part of the subject's care and whose contact with the subject averaged four hours/day for 20 days. The subject asked 119 direct questions which appraised threat (a mean frequency of three to five questions/day over the course of hospitalization). On days immediately prior to each of three major treatment procedures, the subject asked 11-18 questions. Results show that 41% of the total questions were related to threat of physical pain, 36% related to threat of treatment complications, 16% to threat to mobility, and 7% to threat to appearance.

357. Peters, B. M. School-aged children's beliefs about causality of illness: A review of the literature. Maternal-Child Nursing Journal, 1978, 7(3), 143-154.

Consistent throughout the literature related to school-aged children's concepts of causality of illness is the child's belief that illness results from human behavior. The ill child's behavior (particularly misbehavior) is more frequently cited as causing illness than the behavior of other persons. Such beliefs were reported to persist in spite of explanations to the child about the true causal factors. The tendency to relate illness to human action has been noted by several researchers to decrease with increasing age. Other investigators found the tendency to assign the same causal factor to all illnesses to decrease with increasing age. Both trends have been interpreted as evidence of cognitive development which is demonstrated by the child's movement from the subjectivity of precausal cognition toward the greater objectivity of adult causal reasoning. There is evidence that children often misinterpret the intent behind treatment of illness, and view it as hostile or punitive. There is some indication that although children seem to understand the therapeutic purpose of treatment procedures, they frequently question the motives of those administering treatments.

358. Peterson, C., & Bullerman, L. Preop visits--for little people. AORN Journal, 1971, 14(5), 71-73.

This report discusses the effects of a study conducted by a group of senior nursing students on the effect of the preoperative visitation and postoperative recovery. From their sample of some 30 cases, they found that the anxiety, fear and resulting pain experienced by children visited preoperatively was significantly lower than in those who did not receive this service. Case studies are presented to illustrate these findings.

359. Peterson, L. The use of a self-control procedure to minimize pain and anxiety in hospitalized children (Doctoral dissertation, University of Utah, 1978). Dissertation Abstracts International, 1978, 39(6-B), 3000.

The effectiveness of a combination of three behavioral coping techniques (relaxation, distractive imagery, and comforting self-talk) was compared with a minimal preparation technique and a filmed modeling technique in reducing children's adverse reactions to elective tonsillectomies. Sixty-six children ages 2.5 to 10.5 and their parents were treated in small groups using minimal information preparation and one of the following procedures: control (minimal preparation only), self-coping, filmed modeling, or self-coping plus filmed modeling. Their reactions to hospitalization and elective tonsillectomies were evaluated using several observational, behavioral, physiological, and self-report techniques. Observational results from the laboratory technician who drew blood and the nurse who gave the preoperative injection indicated children receiving coping plus modeling techniques were most calm and cooperative during invasive procedures. Observational measures from the parent and the observer indicated that the coping procedures were more effective in reducing children's anxiety after surgery than modeling or control procedures. There were marginally significant results indicating that behavioral/physiological data were better for chidlren in the coping groups. Finally, parent self-ratings and ratings of the hospital experience indicated that parents in the coping groups felt calmer, more competent, and rated the experience as better than parents in the other groups. Results are attributed to increased emotional support and feelings of control over the situation for children and parents in the coping condition groups.

360. Peterson, L., & Ridley-Johnson, R. Pediatric hospital response to survey on prehospital preparation for children. Journal of Pediatric Psychology, 1980, 5(1), 1-7.

A survey of all nonchronic care pediatric hospitals in the United States revealed that the majority (70%) of the hospitals offer prehospital preparation to both the parent and the child. A variety of preparation techniques are currently in use, including a narrative explanation of the hospital experience, printed materials such as story books, films, puppet shows, and other therapeutic techniques. The greatest limitation in the preoperative programs appeared to be the relatively low percentage of children served by existing programs. Suggestions regarding the reasons behind this widespread implementation of prehospital preparation and possible improvements in future preparation programs are offered.

361. Petrillo, M Preparing children and parents for hospitalization and treatment. Pediatric Annals, 1972, 1(3), 24-41.

It seems unnecessary today in this age of enlightenment regarding child care practices to find children admitted to hospitals on the pretext of attending pleasurable activities or without any prior knowledge of the event. Medical personnel with only the briefest experience in a pediatric setting can document the fact that these situations still regularly occur. This article discusses the preparation of children and their parents for hospitalization and treatment in order to equip the child with the tools for coping with fear, and to help both the child and his family come to terms with painful events and procedures.

362. Petrillo, M., & Sanger, S. Emotional care of hospitalized children: An environmental approach. Philadelphia: J. B. Lippincott Company, 1980.

In working with children, parents and staff, the authors have evolved, through trial and error, a comprehensive program that applies theory to improving the lot of children who become hospitalized. In seeing the effects of hospitalization on children, it was observed that there was a need for an explicit guide-in-depth of just how to deal with the common problems: (a) of the effects of severe stress, and (b) of everyday coping abilities of children and parents. This exposition is divided into major areas that coalesce into a health-promoting milieu. These areas are: a general knowledge of growth and development, the forces of family and culture, human reactions to stress, loss and separation. Also, preventive approaches that have the effect of minimizeing trauma to children and their families are given in the form of actual protocols.

363. Pidgeon, V. A. Functions and content of verbal contacts initiated by disadvantaged and advantaged preschool children with adults in a hospital (Doctoral dissertation, University of Pittsburgh, 1974). Dissertation Abstracts International, 1974, 34(10-B), 5041.

This was a comparative study of the functions and content of verbal contacts initiated with adults by disadvantaged and advantaged hospitalized preschool children. The subjects were 24 moderately ill children ranging in age from three to six years. Twelve of the subjects were from welfare families and 12 from families considered to be advantaged on the basis of the fathers' occupations and presence of both parents in the home. There were no significant differences in the number of verbal contacts initiated in each of the functional categories by disadvantaged and advantaged children. Disadvantaged children were found to express fewer wants for services and more wants for the attention of adults and to verbalize less about their parents. Analysis of the specific types of verbal contacts and their frequencies are also discussed by the author.

364. Pidgeon. V. A. Functions and content of verbal contacts initiated by disadvantaged and advantaged preschool children with adults in a hospital. Maternal-Child Nursing Journal, 1974, 3(4, Monograph #3).

The author studied the nature and frequency of verbal contacts with adults by 24 hospitalized preschool-age children as a function of socioeconomic status. Subjects were seven girls and five boys from welfare families (disadvantaged group); and five girls and seven boys from intact middle- to upper-class families (advantaged group). Verbal interactions of children with adults were observed and recorded verbatim in structured and unstructured situations. The major findings were that: (a) advantaged and disadvantaged children did not differ significantly in the frequency of verbal contacts with adults; (b) most of the verbal contacts (60%) were information requests; approximately 20% expressed wants or requested adult action; 1% related to the experience of feelings; and (c) disadvantaged children talked less about their parents and expressed more wants for adult attention, while advantaged children verbalized more wants for hospital services. It is concluded that both advantaged and disadvantaged hospitalized children can be articulate and verbal in expressing wants, thought, and feelings and in obtaining responses from adults.

365. Pike, N. In hospital--3: The child's view. Nursing Mirror, 1975, 140(19), 67-68.

Over the past 50 years there has been an increasing awareness of the physical, educational, and social needs of children in hospital. This article discusses the views of hospital life held by a group of children, and several conclusions are presented: (1) If a child had visited a hospital, invaribaly the first impression was "the smell"; (2) The preparation of planned admission appears to have improved the outlook on hospitalization; (3) Medicines and injections were the main causes of distress and fear; and (4) Children whose parents visited them frequently were much happier and more contented. The emotional needs of children in hospital are examined.

366. Pill, R. The sociological aspects of the case-study sample. In M. Stacey (Ed.), Hospitals, children and their families: The report of a pilot study. London: Routledge & Kegan Paul, Ltd., 1970, 85-126.

The evidence presented in this chapter relates to a sample of children who entered one of two hospitals for tonsillectomy and adenoidectomy. Certain problems arose in the course of the research. These stemmed mainly from young children being the subject of study and the environment in which they were being observed. The fact that the behavior of young children was being studied raised the question as to how such behavior was susceptible to sociological analysis and to what extent young children are suitable subjects for sociological research. The data collected by interviews of the child patients' mothers in their own home before the child went to hospital and by observation of the child in whichever of the two hospitals studied he was admitted to is presented and discussed.

367. Pill, R. Health careers and competence: Aspects of behaviour on a children's ward. Social Science and Medicine, 1976, 10(2), 105-111.

Hitherto the literature on patient behaviour in hospital has emphasized environmental variables in the case of adults and psychological variables in the case of children. It is assumed that behaviour on the ward will be affected by the individual's definition of the situation and his interpersonal skills, which will reflect his past experiences. Hardly any studies, however, deal with the way that pre-patient roles and experiences are carried over into the in-patient phase and, in particular, how variation in patterns of illness and treatment might influence behaviour. It is argued here that health status is an important variable which restricts the range and type of interaction possible and hence the opportunity to acquire appropriate interpersonal skills. This approach is explored using data from a sample of children in an orthopaedic ward who varied in age and health status and who were found to vary in the amount of interaction that took place, the tactics they employed and their relative success.

368. Pill, R. The long-stay child patient: The problems. Nursing Times, 1977, 73(27), supplement, 89-92.

In any discussion of the long-stay child patient, the problems he faces and the problems he poses for the health professionals who deal with him, the question of definition becomes crucial. It is argued that any definition relying on passage of time will be inadequate as it is simply a crude indicator of other, more complex social and treatment variables which need separate consideration. Particular categories of children are identified as being at risk of becoming long-stay patients and the problems of providing adequate care for them in a hospital setting are discussed.

369. Pill, R. Status and career: A sociological approach to the study of child patients. In D. Hall and M. Stacey (Eds.), Beyond separation: Further studies of children in hospital. London: Routledge & Kegan Paul, Ltd., 1979, 128-154.

This chapter demonstrates how consideration of the individual child should be extended to take into account sociological concepts of health status and social career. The concept of career embraces both the objective features of movement through a set of situations (as from home to hospital to home) and the subjective meaning attached to such movement. The categorization in terms of health-status and treatment-career variables highlights a neglected group of child patients, namely the recurrent admissions. The implicit dichotomy of the long-stay versus the short-stay patient tends to obscure the fact that a great many children have a history of admissions. Little is known about the long-term psychological effects of repeated admissions and there is no evidence to suggest that this pattern is any less damaging to a child's mental health than a stay involving months. The concept of health status and the career perspective have much wider implications. An attempt is made to relate them within the wider context of socialization theory and to indicate their potential with regard to other categories involved with the child, particularly parents. These concepts are not exclusively child focused, however, since it seems possible to examine the interaction between parents and doctors using their definitions of the child's health status as an explanatory tool.

370. Plank, E. N. Emotional care as a priority: Approaches to implementation. Journal of the Association for the Care of Children in Hospitals, 1974, 3(1), 11-14.

This article discusses the threats hospitalization poses to children, and the emotional care which can be provided by medical staff. Several comments from hospitalized children are presented and discussed.

371. Plank, E. N. The child before operation. Hexagon, 1976, 4(2), 1-8.

This article discusses the role of the child life worker in preparing the child for different hospital procedures. Emergency admission, preplanned surgery, collective preparation, ambulatory surgery, and preparation of the ward are explored briefly with discussion of the role of the child life worker in preoperative preparation in each. Case examples are presented to illustrate the author's points. A list of books that can be used directly with children when preparing them for surgery is also included.

372. Pomarico, C., Marsh, K., & Doubrava, P. Hospital orientation for children. AORN Journal, 1979, 29(5), 864-870, 875.

This article describes an orientation program implemented at a suburban general hospital in Connecticut. The objectives of the program were to: (1) decrease children's fears and anxieties about hospitals through a formalized orientation program; (2) provide a monthly tour and slide presentation to disseminate information about the hospital to potential health care recipients; and (3) increase the pediatric nurses' awareness of the emotional needs of children related to illness and hospitalization. Since the start of this orientation program a year and a half ago, the staff generally agrees that the attitudes of both children and parents have improved. Anticipating and relieving the children's fears about hospitalization is better than trying to treat these fears after hospitalization.

373. Popper, B. Children in hospitals report. Journal of the Association for the Care of Children in Hospitals, 1975, 3(3), 16.

In 1972 a group of parents in Massachusetts formed Children in Hospitals, Inc. to educate parents and health care professionals to the need for continued and ample family contact when either children or their parents are hospitalized. Joined by many health care professionals, the group has encouraged hospitals to adopt flexible visiting policies and to provide living-in accommodations whenever possible. The author of this report, as chairman and co-founder of the group, has repeatedly encountered certain questions and attitudes from parents and professionals. These questions and their answers are presented to health-care professionals to increase their awareness of some of the feelings of parents and staff.

374. Porter, L. S. On the importance of activity. Maternal-Child Nursing Journal, 1973, 2(2), 85-91.

This article attempts to convey the importance of activity in the overall growth and development of infants and children. Activity is discussed as a positive factor enhancing the life process. Findings from motion studies which strongly support the assertion that there is a substantial relationship between activity and infants' rate of growth and development are presented, and a study conducted on hospitalized preschool children which examines the problem of movement restraint is described.

375. Post, S. Commentary. Canadian Nurse, 1977, 73(11), 44-45.

Chldren admitted to hospital are plunged into unfamiliar and frightening surroundings, separated from their family, and subjected to intrusive, often painful, procedures. Without support and assistance in coping with the stress of these experiences, some of them are slow to recover, exhibit developmental regression, develop fears of abandonment and mutilation, or exhibit emotional problems at home and at school after they leave hospital. Despite the fact that for the past twenty years we have had quantities of research and documentation regarding the emotional and developmental responses of children to illness and hospitalization, the policies, routines, and environments of many of our pediatric units have changed little in the past decade. Many changes have been identified which could improve the hospitalization experience for children. Most of these do not require new legislation or large amounts of money but, rather, involve changes in attitudes, policies, and the recognition that we cannot model or transfer traditions and policies established for adult units to children's units. Children have special needs and problems that we must not continue to ignore. Some of these special needs are: (1) visiting; (2) play programs; (3) schooling; and (4) information and orientation.

376. Post, S. Trends in peadiatric hospitals (sic). Dimensions in Health Service, 1979, 56(5), 51-53.

This article explores and documents what some of the common practices in children's units in general hospitals are in regard to visiting, play programs, school opportunities and information given to children and their families about hospitalization. A questionnaire was sent to all pediatric units with more than 20 pediatric beds in British Columbia, Alberta, Manitoba, Quebec, Newfoundland, Northwest Territories, and Yukon. The 125 questionnaires sent were addressed to the hospital administrator. There was an overall response of 75 percent. This article reports some of the findings from this survey.

377. Powazek, M., Goff, J. R., Schyving, J., & Paulson, M. A. Emotional reactions of children to isolation in a cancer hospital. Journal of Pediatrics, 1978, 92(5), 834-837.

Emotional reactions of 123 hospitalized children and their mothers were evaluated during standard isolation with limited visitation and during peninsula isolation with visitation only through glass partitions. Self-report surveys and behavioral observations by nurses indicated that (1) patients and parents in both isolation facilities had overall high levels of hospital-related anxiety and depression which varied with the patient's chronologic age; and (2) parents of preschool children had more negative opinions toward peninsula isolation than did parents of older children. These results confirm the need for psychologically supportive programs for the families of children being treated for catastrophic diseases.

378. Powell, B. S. Laughter and healthing: The uses of humor in hospitals treating children. Journal of the Association for the Care of Children in Hospitals, 1974, 3(2), 10-16.

Most people take a dim view of humor in hospitals. It seems incongruous to mention humor and hospitals in the same breath. Yet humor is part of the human condition and has many positive uses. Although it is tempered by fears children have, it does not cease to exist when children enter the hospital. This paper, presented at the Ninth Annual Conference of the Association for the Care of Children in Hospitals, 1974, discusses how children use humor in hospital settings and how hospital personnel might encourage positive uses of humor among patients.

379. Prout, A. Review of Beyond separation: Further studies of children in hospital by D. Hall and M. Stacey. Sociological Review, 1980, 28(2), 447-448.

This is an important collection of research reports presenting not only new empirical findings but also the beginnings of a more sophisticated theoretical framework and a series of important practical recommendations. The collection is a follow-up to an earlier work by M. Stacey, but goes much further in both its conceptualization and the range and detail of its empirical evidence. There are, however, many familiar objects of concern, the central one being the suffering experienced by some children when hospitalized. This is an important book which presents new data and challenging analyses, and, like all good research, it creates as well as answers questions. It will no doubt prove to be essential reading for medical sociologists.

380. Prugh, D. G. Children's reactions to illness, hospitalization, and surgery. In A. M. Freedman and H. I. Kaplan (Eds.), The child: His psychological and cultural development: I. Normal development and psychological assessment. New York: Atheneum, 1972, 181-194.

This article describes the physical, psychological, and social factors which determine the child's adaptive reaction to illness. Disturbed childhood reactions to hospitalization, acute or chronic illness, surgery, handicaps, and terminal illness are examined, and guidelines are presented for the treatment and prevention of these adverse reactions.

381. Prugh, D. G. One of the pieces: Respect for the cultural heritage of the hospitalized child. Journal of the Association for the Care of Children in Hospitals, 1975, 4(2), 1-8.

This keynote address for the Ninth Annual meeting of the Association for the Care of Children in Hospitals focuses on the cultural heritage of the hospitalized child and his family. Several case examples of situations in which respect for the cultural heritage of the hospitalized child and his family had to form a vital part of the approach to diagnosis and treatment are presented and discussed. The implications for pediatric hospital programs are examined.

382. Prugh, D. G., & Eckhardt, L. O. Stages and phases in the response of children and adolescents to illness and injury. In B. W. Camp (Ed.), Advances in behavioral pediatrics: A research manual. Greenwich, Connecticut: JAI Press, 1980, 181-194.

Illness or injury of a serious nature can cause a major disruption in the child's or adolescent's normal phase of growth and development. The individual's genetic endowment, his constitutional characteristics, his developmental capacities, and the nature of his past experiences, including experience with illness, all contribute to his capacity to adapt to such an experience. This adaptive capacity, the degree of noxious stimuli, and the current circumstances, including the family's response, influence the degree of stressful significance and the adaptive outcome. The author of this chapter concludes that the concept of stages or sequential phases in the responses of parents and children to hospitalization, illness, injury, and other catastrophic experiences deserves greater emphasis in pediatric clinical and training programs.

383. Quinby, S., & Bernstein, N. R. Identity problems and the adaptation of nurses to severely burned children. American Journal of Psychiatry, 1971, 128(1), 58-63.

Caring for burned children presents a difficult challenge to the personal and professional identity of nurses. The authors studied the adjustments of new nurses in the field--their initial idealized expectations, their conflict between these goals and reality, and their resolution of this conflict. The nurses realized the unreality of their initial goals and gained a maturity that enabled them to better help the children and to enhance their own self-esteem.

384. Quinton, D., & Rutter, M. Early hospital admissions and later disturbances of behaviour: An attempted replication of Douglas' findings. Developmental Medicine and Child Neurology, 1976, 18(4), 447-459.

The investigators examined data from two epistemiological studies with 1,279 ten-year-olds from the Isle of Wight and 1,689 ten-year-olds from an inner-London borough to investigate J. W. Douglas' findings on the effect of early childhood hospitalizations on later delinquent behavior. This study confirms Douglas' findings that single hospital admissions of children for up to a week carry no increased risk of later emotional or behavioral disturbance. The study also confirms Douglas' finding that repeated hospital admissions are significantly associated with disturbance in later childhood. The association probably applies to both emotional and conduct disorders, is most marked in the case of children from disadvantaged homes, and it may well reflect a causal influence. The validity of the findings is strengthened by the fact that detailed psychiatric assessments gave rise to much the same findings as did teacher questionnaire scores. However, in both cases, repeated hospital admissions were associated with only a small minority of disorders and accounted for little of the variance in children's behavior.

385. Rae, W. A. Hospitalized latency-age children: Implications for psychosocial care. Journal of the Association for the Care of Children in Hospitals, 1981, 9(3), 59-63.

The purpose of this article is to explore some of the common roadblocks to psychosocial growth that impinge upon the development of mastery, body image, cognitive understanding, and family relationships of hospitalized latency-age children. Potential benefits of hospitalization as well as some guidelines for the care of these children are enumerated.

386. Rae, W. A., & Stieber, D. A. Plant play therapy: Growth through growth. Journal of Pediatric Psychology, 1976, 1(4), 18-20.

Having a hospitalized child care for plants is presented as a method through which the child can be helped to adjust to the hospital. The child becomes in this way a caregiver to the plant, can role play "medical" procedures with it, and can use the plant to symbolize growth, healing, and the constructive resolution of parent-separation fears.

387. Rappazzo, J. A. Psychoesthetic environmental design for pediatric care facilities. Journal of the Association for the Care of Children in Hospitals, 1980, 8(4), 85-93.

This article considers various factors in pediatric care facility designs. A number of ideas and recommendations have been suggested on how to keep decoration simple, inexpensive, and yet produce elegant results. One can assume that the medical, allied health, and hospital administrative professions continually strive to improve the form and quality of health care. Meeting the psychological and emotional needs of pediatric patients and hospital personnel through esthetic environmental design is a means of improvement. When considering the welfare and well-being of a child, no expense of time, resources, energy, or imagination can be considered too great.

388. Rasmussen, M., & Murphy, C. M. Hospital admission through a child's eyes. Pediatric Nursing, 1977, 3(3), 43-46.

Admission to hospital happens at least once for every inpatient, and many times for chronically ill children. Nurses tend to view admission as a routine, often inconveniently timed, and rather unimportant process. Although a daily nursing ritual, the admission procedure sets the tone, either positive or negative, for the child's inpatient experience. This article describes nursing actions during this first contact with the family which can get the hospitalization off to a good start. In order to get a child's eye view of the actual admission period, the authors interviewed a dozen hospitalized patients and their parents. The authors conclude that admission procedure should have three objectives: (1) to welcome the child and his parents; (2) to acquaint the family with physical services available, tell them when the physician will arrive to talk with them and to present necessary forms; and (3) to exchange information with the parents regarding the child's care and his need for hospitalization.

389. Resnick, R., & Hergenroeder, E. Children and the emergency room. Children Today, 1975, 4(5), 5-8.

To learn more about children in emergency situations, a pilot study was conducted at the Pediatric Trauma Center of the Children's Medical and Surgical Center, Johns Hopkins Hospital. One hundred children, chosen at random from patients between the ages of three and 13, were surveyed for the study. Information about each child and the injury was taken, and an anecdotal record was kept of the behaviors and verbalization of both the patient and the adult who accompanied him or her. From this study several important concerns were identified that require further consideration. First, although the importance of play to hospitalized children has often been emphasized, meaningful play activities are seldom offered in the emergency room. The opportunity for play in this stressful environment is a vital part of care and should be offered whenever possible. A second area concerns the "psychological" treatment of parents, which may be as important as the medical treatment of the child-patient. Blank policies which ask all parents to remain in the waiting area can result in much unnecessary anxiety for the child. Third, children reacted more positively when explanations were given prior to treatment. Many children who were shown sutures, dressings, scissors and tape before treatment was begun, and who were given as complete an explanation of their use as they could understand, appeared more calm once the "mysteries" of the emergency room had been revealed. Fourth, it is vitally important that emergency room staff members be included in pediatric conferences, meetings, training workshops, etc. Better communications among those knowledgeable in child development, pediatrics and emergency room care can benefit both staff and patient. Finally, more basic research in the area of children's reactions to emergency treatment is needed to improve the care of children in this hospital situation.

390. Rickard, K., & Farnum, S. Food for fun and thought: Nutrition education in a children's hospital. Journal of the American Dietetic Association, 1974, 65(3), 294-297.

Patients in James Whitcomb Riley Hospital for Children and their families had an opportunity to learn more about nutrition through "Food for Fun and Thought" projects in which they participated in educational cookery. These projects were planned so that elementary school age children (ages seven to twelve) had a positive, successful, and creative learning experience in the hospital, often a place of trauma. The most successful projects included cooking which used gross and fine motor skills and a game as a reinforcing agent for nutrition learning. The children used various social and intellectual skills throughout the cooking and game. The emphasis was on helping the child become emotionally ready to participate, planning experiences which actively involved the child, and structuring the influences around the project so that the child was continually in a positive learning situation.

391. Riddle, I. Communicative behaviors of hospitalized school age children with binocular bandages. Maternal-Child Nursing Journal, 1972, 1(4), 291-354.

The author studied five schoolchildren who had adequate vision for activities of daily living prior to hospitalization. Four had sustained traumatic eye injuries; one had a retinal detachment. Data was collected through observation and interview. Verbal and nonverbal behavior and interpersonal encounters were analyzed. It was found that subjects were quiet, polite, and generally unresponsive to indirect questions and comments. Two-thirds of the verbal information volunteered by the five subjects in initial interviews was responsive and represented elaborations upon content introduced by the investigator. It is concluded that school-age children are vulnerable to feelings of interpersonal estrangement.

392. Riddle, I. Nursing intervention to promote body image integrity in children. Nursing Clinics of North America, 1972, 7(4), 651-661.

Health problems often pose serious threats to the developing body image of the infant, child, and adolescent.

Principles of nursing intervention can be derived from body image theory to assist the young in mastering health problems and overcoming body image threats. Principles are, by their nature, general guides to nursing intervention. It is in the application of principles in the actual process of care that the sensitivity and creativity of the nurse are manifested. Some of these principles and the role of nursing intervention are discussed in this article.

393. Riddle, I. Caring for children with bandaged eyes. ANA Clinical Sessions, San Francisco, 1974. New York: Appleton-Century-Crofts, 1975, 99-105.

In order to help a child realize the goal of psychosocial relaxation while his eyes are bandaged, his nursing care plan must take into account the interpersonal effects of his bandages. The plan must specify measures to counteract the subjective effects of visual deprivation and must ensure interpersonal continutiy for the child within the caring process.

394. Riddoch, M. Children in hospital in Wales: Final report of the working party on children in hospital in Wales. Nursing Times, 1973, 69(8), 278-279.

The working party has identified problems which exist not only in Wales; it has obtained information from many parts of Britain and has made excellent suggestions in considerable detail for improving facilities and care. In a report reviewed in this article, the working party found deficiencies in accommodation, staffing and supplementary facilities in children's wards and departments. Suggestions for dealing with these problems are also reviewed.

395. Rigg, C. A., & Fisher, R. C. Is a separate adolescent ward worthwhile? American Journal of Disease of Children, 1971, 122, 489-493.

In an attempt to ascertain whether a separate ward for adolescents in a hospital is worthwhile, detailed questionnaires were sent to the medical and nursing staff of hospitals with adolescent programs previously surveyed by the authors. Some of these hospitals had separate adolescent wards and some did not. Sixteen of them were then visited personally by the investigators, who examined the facilities and interviewed both staff and patients. For comparative purposes adolescents in four hospitals without adolescent programs were also interviewed. The consensus of the medical and nursing staff, and the patients, was that a separate adolescent ward is worthwhile.

396. Ritchie, J. Body image changes following amputation in an adolescent girl. Maternal-Child Nursing Journal, 1972, 1(1), 39-46.

This article discusses the case of a thirteen-and-a-half year old girl who was admitted to the hospital for an above-knee amputation. The girl was admitted to hospital two days prior to her scheduled surgery date, and was referred to the child psychiatrist on the day prior to surgery. The referral was made because of concerns with her angry and hostile reactions to the pending surgery. She had refused to talk to the residents or to answer their questions, and had become angry with her own surgeon. After surgery the girl experienced depression and phantom limb feeling in the leg which had been amputated. Steps undertaken to restore the patient's ego functioning with respect to body image change are discussed.

397. Ritchie, J. Fantasy in communicating concerns about body integrity. Maternal-Child Nursing Journal, 1972, 1(2), 117-126.

That separation, body integrity, and intrusion are major concerns of hospitalized pre-school children is well recognized. How the child communicates these concerns or can be helped to master them has been less than adequately described. It is the purpose of this paper to describe one hospitalized child's utilization of fantasy in communication and mastery of separation and body integrity.

398. Ritter, F. L., & Linzing, K. M. B. FPO--For parents only. Journal of the Association for Care of Children in Hospitals, 1980, 9(2), 31-34.

Play therapists in a pediatric institution are seen as child advocates. However, if they are to grow within the field of pediatric medicine and continue to meet the changing needs of the patients, their role must be extended. Working with the parent(s) is an extension of working for the child. This article describes a program for parents only (FPO) at The Children's Hospital of Philadelphia. The meetings are conducted by play therapists who act as facilitators to develop a support system among the parents, and who apply the very techniques used in play therapy sessions with children.

399. Robertson, J. Young children in hospital (2nd edition). London: Tavistock Publications Limited, 1970.

In the ten years following the Platt Report, many improvements have occurred in the management of children's wards, especially in the English-speaking countries. A number of publications have appeared which deal mainly with the practical implications of a concept of care which seeks to safeguard the emotional well-being of young patients, with the responses of children and parents to better facilities, and with the problems thrown up by more enlightened pediatric practice. In preparing the second edition, the author allows the simple statement on mental health considerations stated in the first edition to remain unchanged, while adding a Postscript with particular reference to the unique contribution of an informed public opinion mobilized to hasten the implementation of the Platt Report. Some consideration is also given to the substantial obstacles that still stand in the way of achieving optimal care of the young child in hospital.

400. Robertson, J., & Robertson, J. Substitute mothering. Nursing Times, 1973, 69(47), 1611-1614.

Twelve years after its modest beginnings, the National Association for the Welfare of Children in Hospital has good reason to be pleased with the part it has played in obtaining the high degree of implementation of the Platt Report which now exists--including unrestricted visiting in most children's wards, and a growing number of wards where mothers can stay with their children. Throughout the first decade the main focus of activity has understandably been upon the concerned and articulate mother and her hospitalized child, because it is these mothers who bring to attention most forcefully the stresses that various restrictions can cause to both mother and child. The authors believe that we should now consider that substantial part of the hospital population which has so far received much less of the attention. There are many young children in short-stay and long-stay wards who have insufficient contact with their mothers. If a young child loses the care of his mother it is essential that his experience of mothering be continued in order to safeguard the child's normal development. Therefore, if a child in a short- or long-term ward has insufficient contact with the mother the onus rests upon the hospital to substitute as well as possible for the loss of her care.

401. Robertson, M., & Barford, F. Story-making in psychotherapy with a chronically ill child. <u>Psychotherapy: Theory, Research, and Practice</u>, 1970, <u>7</u>(2), 104-107.

Child psychotherapy seeks through play procedures to reinforce reality situations. Chronically ill children who are immobilized in hospital settings have little opportunity, except in directed play or fantasy, to act out the psychic problems connected with their situation. As a consequence, story-making psychotherapy offers the child a means of acting out in fantasy those feelings which he could not express in reality. Use of stories written specifically for children in hospitals (1) results in more socialization and a more vivid reality as the child begins to master his feelings by overt expression of them, and (2) enables the child to act out in fantasy the feelings which he was unable to act out in reality. This article presents several case studies demonstrating how this form of psychotherapy can be of help in treating those faced with the traumatic experiences of hospitalization.

402. Robinson, D. The social milieu. In M. Stacey (Ed.), Hospitals, children and their families: The report of a pilot study. London: Routledge & Kegan Paul, Ltd., 1970, 14-54.

Although a good deal of attention has been paid to child patients, their behavior, their needs and their treatment, little is known systematically about the attitudes and behavior of their parents. The survey upon which this chapter is based was one facet of a project concerned with social and psychiatric aspects of the welfare of children in hospital. The survey, however, was in no way designed to study either children or hospitals. It was, rather, a study of certain aspects of the process whereby a child moves from his home environment into the hospital system and back again. The implementation of official policy, the process of hospitalization, visiting, living-in, attitudes, and the differences between a hospital and non-hospital sample are discussed.

403. Robinson, G. C., & Clarke, H. F. Day care surgery. In G. C. Robinson and H. F. Clarke (Eds.), The hospital care of children: A review of contemporary issues. Oxford: Oxford University Press, 1980, 116-130.

Day care surgery usually refers to a hospital service which allows admission and discharge on the day of surgery. It requires general anaesthesia and is reserved for elective operative procedures. The patient receives the same hospital treatment with regard to care, safety, and medical records as would an inpatient. It is not synonymous with outpatient surgery, and it is unwise to anaesthetize outpatients except for minor operations unless there is an organized day care surgical unit. This chapter reviews some of the advantages of day care surgery. There are three reasons for promoting this form of care. First, it minimizes emotional disturbance because it reduces the separation of the young child and parent to a few hours. Second, it reduces the risk of hospital-acquired infection. Third, the cost is significantly lower than when performed on an inpatient basis, without compromising the quality of care.

404. Robinson, G. C., & Clarke, H. F. Family centered care in hospital. In G. C. Robinson and H. F. Clarke (Eds.), The hospital care of children: A review of contemporary issues. Oxford: Oxford University Press, 1980, 68-89.

This chapter reviews the historical development of family centered care, its rationale and scope, different applications in health care settings, and its acceptance by users and consumers. The authors point out that there has been a gradual shift from an institutional to a family centered philosophy of care during the past two decades. The initial emphasis was on the psychological needs of the child and family with the introduction of open visiting, parent participation, and play and education programs to normalize the life of the child in hospital. More recently, the impact of these ideas upon the family and the hospital staff has been recognized. It is anticipated that the wider preparation of children for hospital experiences and the special concern for vulnerable children, together with the redefinition of professional roles and retraining, will combine to further humanize the stay in hospital of children.

405. Roper-Hall, G. Reaction of children to hospitalization for strabismus surgery. British Orthoptic Journal, 1970, 27, 100-107.

The effect of hospitalization on children can be an accumulative psychological trauma. By shortening the stay in hospital and encouraging the parents and staff to produce a system as near to that in the child's home as possible, these effects can be reduced to a minimum. This report outlines a system developed for the ophthalmic ward at the Royal Berkshire Hospital. Parents have the choice of either visiting at frequent intervals or staying overnight. A survey of this method showed that the parents seem happy with this method, and that the children, as the figures show, seem to be largely unaffected by the experience of hospitalization.

406. Rose, M. H. The effects of hospitalization on the coping behaviors of children. In M. V. Batey (Ed.), Communicating nursing research. Boulder, Colorado: Western Interstate Commission for Higher Education, 1972, 115-126.

Hospitalization, a stressful experience encountered by many children, has been the topic of many articles and books; however, relatively few systematic studies have been done in this area. Unlike the present study, most of the studies which have been done were based on the assumption that hospitalization and separation from mother were psychologically harmful, producing immediate and possible long-term undesirable changes in children's behavior. An implicit assumption underlying these studies seems to be that all children and families had the same limited capacity with which to deal with stress. The propositions underlying this study are that most children have the capacity to cope with and develop from stressful situations and thus changes seen in behavior during hospitalization will be temporary. The purpose of the study was to investigate how children cope with the experience of hospitalization. The results of the study demonstrated that children showed similar changes in behavior in the hospital, even though the magnitude of change was different from child to child. Following hospitalization the children largely reverted back to their prehospital behavior. It is proposed that the way in which the children changed during hospitalization was dependent in large measure on the nature of the hospital experience and organization, while the magnitude of change was influenced by the children's coping capacities and the interaction between individual children and persons with whom they came in contact.

407. Rose, M. H. Response to critique. In M. V. Batey (Ed.), Communicating nursing research. Boulder, Colorado: Western Interstate Commission for Higher Eduation, 1972, 132-133.

This short response answers the critique of the author's paper "The effects of hospitalization on the coping behaviors of children," made by B. J. Hadley in this same volume. While the author feels that the criticism concerning the theoretical base of the study is valid, she defends her use of parametric statistics and the interpretations based on the data. In regard to her conclusions, they were based very heavily on the qualitative data and need to be checked through further study. She believes very strongly that we have been looking too closely just at the children's behaviors, and not closely enough at the behaviors of the people about them.

408. Roskies, E., & Bedard, P. Emergency hospitalization of young children: Some neglected psychological considerations. Medical Care, 1975, 13(7), 570-581.

In spite of the fact that emergency admission is the most common form of hospitalization for young children, as well as containing the greatest potential for trauma, almost no reference has been made to it in the psychological literature on pediatric hospitalization. To explore the theoretical and practical feasibility of research in this area, a pilot study was designed to investigate the reactions of a sample of children, parents, and staff to the first six hours of emergency hospitalization, compared with those of a similar sample to elective admission. Sixteen children (eight in each group) aged 11 to 48 months were selected on a time-sample basis from the patient population of a large, metropolitan, pediatric hospital and were followed by trained observers using a specially designed observation schedule. The results indicated that, as expected, emergency does constitute an even greater stress for children, parents, and staff than the already stressful situation of elective admission. In both conditions, however, the results were more complex and more disturbing than anticipated. The implications of these findings, as well as suggestions for further research, are discussed.

409. Roskies, E., Mongeon, M., & Fagnon-Lefebvre, B. Increasing maternal participation in the hospitalization of young children. Medical Care, 1978, 16(9), 765-777.

The study described here sought to increase mothers' participation in their children's hospitalization by overcoming some of the psychological barriers believed to exist. The mothers of 48 children aged one to five, to be admitted for elective surgery to a large, metropolitan pediatric hospital, constituted the primary sample and were divided into experimental and control groups. Mothers in the experiemntal group had an extra half-hour session in a pre-admission interview focusing on visiting, and specific suggestions were made about frequency and timing of visits, as well as the role of the mother during her visits. During the experimental period weekly meetings were held with the nursing staff to enlist their support for this change in visiting patterns. Results indicate that duration of visits, timing of visits, and behavior during them were all significantly modified for the experimental group of mothers. In contrast, the nurses did not significantly change their relationship with the mothers or the children. Clinical possibilities and limitations of such a program are discussed.

410. Rossman, P. G., & Miller, D. The effects of social prejudice on hospitalized adolescents. American Journal of Psychiatry, 1973, 130(9), 1029-1031.

The authors describe an outbreak of intragroup prejudice on an adolescent service. The disturbance was traced to patient anxiety over prejudice against the mentally ill, as exemplified in a national event, the withdrawal of Senator Thomas Eagleton as a candidate for Vice-President. The role of social prejudice as a source of anxiety and disturbed behavior within a hospital setting is stressed.

411. Rubin, M. The therapeutic use of separation during hospitalization: An alternative to pediatric rooming-in. In M. Duffey, E. H. Anderson, B. S. Bergersen, M. Lohr, and M. H. Rose (Eds.), Current concepts in clinical nursing, Volume III. St. Louis: C. V. Mosby Company, 1971, 99-105.

Most children have relatively healthy relationships with their mothers. Rooming-in during hospitalization or at least unlimited visiting, with support and help from the nurse, will help these children and their mothers grow during the crisis of illness and hospitalization. Exceptions to the rule indicate that separation of a special type may be necessary in order for the experience to provide growth. Planned separation does allow for exceptions--that all children are not better off with their own parent(s). A structured and realistic separation is not inevitably traumatic; separation is available as a relieving and therapeutic tool.

412. Rumfelt, J. J. M. How five year old children perceive the role of the nurse. Maternal-Child Nursing Journal, 1980, 9(1), 13-24.

This article describes a study which had as its purpose the exploration of the five-year-old child's perception of the nurse's role and the discovery of whether this perception differs between children who are in the hospital and those who have never been hospitalized. Results indicated that the children viewed the nurse as a person who could be identified by apparel: namely, a white uniform, white shoes, a cap and a pin. The perceptions of the nursery school children without prior hospital experience did not differ substantially from those of children who had been hospitalized.

413. Rutkowski, J. A survey of child life programs. Journal of the Association for the Care of Children in Hospitals, 1978, 6(2), 11-16.

The author summarizes questionnaire responses describing 120 programs in pediatric and in general hospitals designed to meet children's emotional needs while they are hospitalized. Such programs are relatively new, offer a variety of services in need of evaluation, and face problems in funding, staffing, space allocation, and coordination with other hospital services.

414. Sadler, J. E., Jr. Coordinated pediatric care through a liaison team. Pediatric Annals, 1972, 1(3), 72-78.

A properly functioning psychiatric liaison team greatly adds to pediatric care by helping to form a composite picture of the child. This paper describes the development of such a team in a pediatric setting, with particular attention to the National Jewish Hospital and Research Center in Denver, Colorado. The specific roles of the team members are outlined and discussion of how this particular unit functions well is presented.

415. Sadler, J. E., Jr. The long-term hospitalization of asthmatic children. Pediatric Clinics of North America, 1975, 22(1), 173-183.

It is with reluctance that most physicians would consider long-term hospitalization of their patients, even those children who have severely chronic asthma. As in all medical treatments, the physician must weigh the potential harmful effects, or risks, of a given treatment against the potential therapeutic gains for the child. With proper care to potential risks of hospitalization, however, there is evidence in favor of long-term hospitalization as a specific treatment tool for asthmatic children. This article reports on the current Pediatrics Behavioral Sciences Program at the National Jewish Hospital and Research Center which provides for the long-term medical and psychologic treatment of children from infancy to adulthood who suffer from chronic intractable asthma.

416. Sauerman, T. H. A guide for dealing with five major life issues of young children (ages 2-7): Death, hospitalization and illness, separation and divorce, new baby, and moving (Doctoral dissertation, Temple University, 1980). Dissertation Abstracts International, 1980, 41(5-A), 1939.

This study is a guide for teachers of children ages two to seven to enable them to assist young children to deal with five major life issues, including hospitalization and illness. In addition to a review of related research and literature, there is an exposition of Piaget's description of the preoperational child and implications for life issues. An extensive investigation of bibliotherapy is followed with guidance for its use in the classroom. Each life issue is dealt with in a separate chapter having two sections: (1) Issues related to the topic are based on a review of resarch. Following each issue the author formulates implications for teachers. (2) Resources are suggested for teachers to use in class under the following headings: Books for Children, Audio-visuals for Children, Classroom Activities, and Visits and Visitors. The chapter dealing with hospitalization and illness contains additional suggestions for teachers who wish to study the topic further under the following headings: Special Programs, Organizations, Ideas for Parent Group Meetings, and Books for Adults. The study concludes that teachers can play an important part in helping young chidlren cope with these difficult life events. Their role is not to shield the children but to support and enable them to grow from the experience.

417. Savedra, M. Coping with pain: Strategies of severely burned children. Maternal-Child Nursing Journal, 1976, 5(3), 197-203.

Nurses and others responsible for the care of the burned child are constantly involved in procedures which inflict pain, attempting to get the child to cooperate in pain producing experiences, and coping with the child's response to pain. While nurses who work with such children expect to experience outbursts from the child, they are often unprepared for the intensity and duration of the child's response. Observations of five children hospitalized with severe burns were taken to determine how a child copes with the intense, seemingly never-ending pain of an extensive burn. All five of the children studied could be classified as active copers, and patterns of coping could be identified for individual children. It would appear from this limited sample that postponement was frequently attempted and was more common than attempting to bypass the pain producing situation. Strategies to reduce threat were also common while devices to divert attention were infrequently used. Creating distance between self and the threat was not physically possible for the severely burned child.

418. Savedra, M. K. The severely burned child: Moving from hospital to home. MCN: American Journal of Maternal Child Nursing, 1977, 2 (4), 220-222.

When the hospital stay of a burned child is relatively brief, little time is needed for the child to prepare psychologically for leaving the hospital. But the child whose stay is lengthy needs considerable time, particularly when her life has been in danger and she has been dependent on others for every aspect of her own care. This article presents a case study of a severely burned school-aged child which illustrates the process entailed in psychological preparation for discharge.

419. Savedra, M. The adolescent in the hospital. In R. T. Mercer (Ed.), Perspectives on adolescent health care. New York: J. B. Lippincott Company, 1979, 172-185.

Illness with hospitalization is not the usual experience for the adolescent. Coming at a time when the youth is dealing with major developmental tasks regarding independence, sexual identity, peer relations, and future job and career goals, it adds an extra stress to an already critical period. Though hospitalization may impede the accomplishment of the developmental tasks, it may also aid in their accomplishment. Whether hospitalization is ultimately a positive or negative experience for the adolescent depends to a large degree on the understanding, interest and sensitive care of the nurse and other members of the health team.

420. Schmeltz, K. An early latency child's use of obsessional ritual to master separation anxiety. Maternal-Child Nursing Journal, 1977, 6(2), 117-134.

It is evident that separation anxiety is an affect that has the potential to arise first in late infancy and to continue throughout early latency. The characteristics of separation anxiety, however, change in each successive stage of the child's development. Rituals and other obsessive-compulsive behaviors are mechanisms which are newly available to the early latency child to deal with threats to the ego. The stressful hospitalization experience may precipitate the resurgence of separation anxiety in early latency. The common denominator between the occurrence of separation anxiety and the use of obsessive behavior is the appearance of each phenomenon as a result of regression to the anal-sadistic level of psychosexual development. Therefore, it is not surprising that an early latency child may deal with the stress of separation anxiety by using obsessional ritual. This article describes the case of a five and one-half year old girl who became involved in repetitive verbalizations that evoked images of home and repetitive structuring of actions to stimulate the maternal milieu. These rituals were used in an attempt to master separation anxiety during hospitalization.

421. Schooley, C. C. Communicating with hospitalized children: The mutal storytelling technique. Journal of Pastoral Care, 1974, 28, 102-111.

Mutual Storytelling invites the child to tell a completely imaginary story to another person. Once the child has related his story, another version of the story is told in return by the second individual (normally a therapist, pastor, chaplain or teacher). This second story aims at reinterpreting the original, seeking to present different alternatives for the outcome or different character models for the main actors. Adaptation of this technique, coupled with a comprehension of the medical experience from the point of view of the child, leads to valuable relationships between support personnel and young patient. Support, hope, and healing can be encouraged and expression of despair, anger, anxiety, and fantasy developed for the hospitalized child.

422. Schowalter, J. E. The utilization of child psychiatry on a pediatric adolescent ward. Journal of the American Academy of Child Psychiatry, 1971, 10(4), 684-699.

Admission reactions of young children to the hospital are well described, but little has been published specifically about adolescent patients. In this paper the author has discussed from the child psychiatry point of view the problems encountered and the approach used since the Yale-New Haven Hospital Adolescent Unit was opened in autumn, 1966. The author stresses the need for pediatrician-child psychiatrist collaboration and the fact that serious illness with hospitalization can represent an especially grave psychological handicap during the developmental stage of adolescence. At present, separate adolescent units in general hospitals remain rare. Their usefulness, however, is no longer doubted, and the burgeoning new field of adolescent medicine will soon have the personnel to make such facilities commonplace. It is in the best tradition of preventive psychiatry for child psychiatrists to take an active part in the development and functioning of these adolescent units.

423. Schowalter, J. E. Working together: Is a children's hospital for children or staff? Journal of the Association for the Care of Children in Hospitals, 1974, 3(1), 3-6.

This speech, given at the Ninth Annual Association for the Care of Children in Hospitals Conference in Chicago, 1974, explores the phenomenon that no matter how much knowledge is available about providing comprehensive care to hospitalized children, only the smallest fraction of the learning is regularly used. To examine why so much less is done than is known how to do, the speaker suggests looking to three areas of interlocking conflict: first, staff reactions as adults to child; second, staff reactions to illness and debility; and third, competition among staff themselves. He believes that in order for professionals to improve their capacity to deliver the level of service that they know how to, these conflicts must be recognized so that conscious action can be taken to diminish their deleterious effect.

424. Schowalter, J. E. Psychological reactions to physical illness and hospitalization in adolescence. Journal of the American Academy of Child Psychiatry, 1977, 16(3), 500-516.

This paper surveys some of the psychoanalytic and psychosomatic literature which comments on the developmental aspects of adolescence and on the impact of bodily illness. Special attention is paid to the influence of debilitation on an adolescent patient's self-esteem and ego-formation. It is suggested that the encouragement of self-care, the facilitation of the appropriate use of signal anxiety, anticipatory mourning and/or denial, as well as education in adaptive skills, are specific measures which are psychologically felicitous for the care of physically ill adolescents.

425. Schowalter, J. E., & Lord, R. D. The hospitalized adolescent. Children, 1971, 18(4), 127-132.

Over the past 20 years, the idea that adolescents need special medical attention has been attracting more and more supporters. This article describes the development of a program of adolescent services which included both inpatient and outpatient care at the Department of Pediatrics at Yale Medical School in 1965. The psychological aspects of the experience are discussed.

426. Schowalter, J. E., & Lord, R. D. On the writings of adolescents in a general hospital ward. Psychoanalytic Study of the Child, 1972, 27, 181-200.

Illness and hospitalization undoubtedly have much psychological impact on adolescents, although studies to date have primarily focused on younger children. The development of separate wards for adolescents has facilitated investigations of this age group. On the Adolescent Unit of the Yale-New Haven Hospital various approaches have been adopted, which serve several purposes, including that of increasing our understanding of patients. One project is the publishing of a ward newspaper, whose writings over a four-year period well reveal many of these adolescents' frequently expressed feelings and concerns. In this article the authors have attempted to outline and highlight them via the following themes: Contradictory Attitudes, Food, Bowel Function, Sexual Differences and Concerns, Anger and Criticism, Basic Danger Situations, Staff, and Going Home.

427. Schultz, N. V. How children perceive pain. Nursing Outlook, 1971, 19(10), 670-673.

This study surveyed the reactions of 74 ten- and eleven-year old boys and girls to hospitalization and pain. The sample was drawn from a public grammar school and consisted of both black and white children. Results showed that 39 of the 74 children had been hospitalized at some time. Previous hospitalization did not seem to have much effect on the children's answers to how they feel when they have pain. Only eight out of the 74 said that when they felt pain they wanted to cry and did. Often the boys answered "brave", but also "nervous" or "afraid." The first answer of "brave" seems to express what nurses and society expect, and the last two constitute a compromise he allows himself --as long as he doesn't cry--because "only babies cry," or "big boys don't cry." The remainder of the article relates these preliminary survey findings to psychological issues related to hospitalization.

428. Schwartz, A. H. Children's concepts of research hospitalization. New England Journal of Medicine, 1972, 287(12), 589-592.

Current concern for legal and ethical aspects of informed consent in children prompted this study of 50 hospitalizations of 36 children, four to 17 years of age, to determine their concepts of the research nature of their hospitalization. In spite of careful preparation, none of the 17 children under and only six of the 19 over the age of 11 showed awareness during admission that their hospitalization had anything to do with research. Five of the six who showed some awareness of research presented symptoms of overwhelming anxiety. This study suggests that even after careful preparation the child subject most often is not aware of the research nature of his hospitalization. It further suggests that only after 11 years of age may a child be aware of being a research subject and that such an awareness may result in overwhelming anxiety.

429. Seegel, V. F. The divorced parent and the hospitalized child: Implications for the hospital staff. Journal of the Association for the Care of Children in Hospitals, 1978, 7(2), 16-18.

This article discusses the potential impact of a child's illness and hospitalization upon the single or divorced parent. Such individuals are seen to be especially vulnerable to stress and in need of the understanding support of hospital staff. Three case studies are presented to illustrate the needs of the parents, the child patients, and other children in the family. The parents' need to maintain relationships with new partners is noted. Group discussions for parents of hospitalized children are viewed as helpful.

430. Seeley, E. F. Coping behavior of an immobilized eight year old. Maternal-Child Nursing Journal, 1973, 2(1), 14-21.

This article describes the coping behavior of an immobilized eight year old girl who was injured at the age of two years in a car accident. The child's behavior in relation to coping with immobilization differed in each of three specific phases of her present eight-day hospitalization: (1) the three-day period prior to immobilization; (2) the initial two-day period of immobilization; and (3) the three-day convalescent phase of hospitalization, during which time she remained continuously immobilized. These three stages are described.

431. Seligman, R. A psychiatric classification system for burned children. American Journal of Psychiatry, 1974, 131(1), 41-46.

The author proposes a system for the classification of burned children designed to identify children's normal and pathological responses to severe burns and to facilitate research into the prevention of serious psychological complications. The classification system has three main categories, consisting of child-related, burn-related, and environment-related items; these are numerically coded in an order that provides a prognostic assessment. The author hopes that this system will permit the identification of patients who are most in need of psychiatric care during their course of treatment.

432. Seligman, R., Macmillan, B. G., & Carroll, S. S. The burned child: A neglected area of psychiatry. American Journal of Psychiatry, 1971, 128(1), 52-57.

Children suffering major burn injury were studied; four case vignettes are presented. Significant factors that emerged included unconscious motivation and early parent loss in some parents of burned children, an unexpected finding. Positive factors for survival were coping mechanisms of denial, withdrawal, splitting of the ego, somatic responses (hypertension, ulcers, and "seizures"), and hope in parents and/or staff. Follow-up revealed better adjustment than anticipated. The authors urge psychiatric involvement in the burned child and offer possible explanations for past neglect.

433. Shade-Zeldow, Y. Attachment and separation: The effects of hospitalization on pediatric patients (Doctoral dissertation, Purdue University, 1976). Dissertation Abstracts International, 1977, 37 (10-B), 5376.

Seventy-five mother-child pairs were the subjects of this study. The children were aged three to 15 years and were hospitalized on a pediatric unit of a general hospital. Pre-hospital and six-week post-hospital ratings of the child's behavior were obtained through completion of the Louisville Behavior Check List (LBCL) by mothers. Similar in-hospital ratings were obtained from nursing staff, using a modified version of the LBCL. The Parent Attitude Research Instrument (PARI) and Mothering Experience Scale (MES) were administered to mothers in an attempt to assess their dependency-fostering attitudes and behaviors. Information was obtained as to each subject's age, sex, number of siblings, presence/absence of surgical intervention, family constellation, length of hospitalization, admission status, and experiences of prior hospitalization. Results showed that age predicted hospital adjustment, with younger children displaying more regression, inhibition, and aggression than their older counterparts. Length of hospitalization predicted hospital adjustment, above and beyond the contribution of age. Children hospitalized for longer periods of time displayed more aggressive behavior. Children admitted on an emergency basis displayed both greater aggressive and inhibitory behavior, above and beyond the effects of pre-hospital adjustment and age. None of the other factors under consideration held significant predictive value in assessing the child's emotional and behavioral response to hospitalization.

434. Shannon, R. M. Use of creativity in coping. Maternal-Child Nursing Journal, 1974, 3(1), 19-30.

This article presents the case study of a five-year-old boy (Billy) hospitalized for cardiac catheterization to determine heart status for surgery. The author discusses this child's behavior under four major categories: (1) self-protection; (2) cognitive mastery; (3) self-expression; and (4) integration of these major areas. The author concludes that Billy was successful in creating a harmonious environment for himself in which he continuously added strength and scope to his ego while dealing with the stress of a life crisis. The predominant factors in Billy's interactions were autonomy and mastery. he consistently repatterned and restructured situations to fulfill his own needs. Billy's innate attributes of temperament and intelligence were complemented by a family environment which encouraged and contributed to those qualities. His developmental age is characterized by elements of creativity. Natural and developmental creative elements were enhanced by circumstantial factors: loss of his mother and intense identification with his father. Continuous strong support and latitude in functioning during the two hospitalizations provided a baseline from which he could function broadly. Billy's flexible use of a wide variety of coping mechanisms in a consistent, reality-oriented manner was identified as creativity.

435. Shope, J. Parental involvement program. Nursing Outlook, 1970, 18(4), 32-34.

A successful parent participation in a hospital rests on several important concepts: that separation of a child from his mother is traumatic, particularly at a time of illness when at least some degree of regression takes place; that a hospital is more therapeutic when it is homelike; that serious illness has implications for the entire family, not just the patient; that a well-informed family is better able to handle anxiety states; and that actively caring for her child under medical and nursing guidance better equips a mother to care for him at home. This article describes a parent participation program at the City of Hope Medical Center, Duarte, California, which involves the health team, the parents, and the sick child.

436. Shaw, J. Volunteers prepare children for surgery through puppet therapy. Modern Hospital, 1970, 114(6), 126-127.

This article describes a program of puppet therapy in effect at Children's Memorial Hospital in Chicago. The puppets prepare children for surgery by a form of role playing. The puppets and props and their amateur puppeteers encourage the child to act out his fears so they will no longer haunt him. The method also acquaints the child with what he is about to experience, so he will know what to expect. The therapy is performed by trained volunteers who are well informed about the operation the child will undergo. Examples of how the therapy has worked to reduce the anxiety of several children are presented.

437. Sheridan, M. S. Children's feelings about the hospital. Social Work in Health Care, 1975, 1(1), 65-70.

The purpose of this article is to identify the painful feelings of hospitalized children and to offer some ways in which a concerned staff can help them cope with these feelings. The following points are discussed as ways to minimize the disturbance of hospitalization: (1) Good communication, so that the patient can share what he wishes; (2) Information, to maximize intellectual mastery and support the healthy coping mechanism; (3) Consideration of feelings, even if the staff cannot do what the patient wishes; and (4) A total milieu in which child and family can feel comfortable, and be assured that everything possible is being done in their behalf.

438. Sheridan, M. S. Talk time for hospitalized children. Social Work, 1975, 20(1), 40-44.

The Talk Time program started at the University of Illinois Hospital focuses on discussion and encourages children to share their fears and fantasies of the hospital experience. The meetings have been useful in the study and diagnosis of the emotional aspects of illness. They have proved effective as well in teaching hospital personnel about pediatric patients and helping them to learn how to listen to the children's needs.

439. Shore, M. F., & Goldston, S. E. Guest editorial. Journal of Pediatric Psychology, 1976, 1(4), 2.

This editorial is a foreword to a special issue of the Journal of Pediatric Psychology which presents some current developments regarding the effects of hospitalization on the mental health of children and their families. The authors argue that although there has been considerable activity focused on the mental health considerations of hospitalization, much remains to be done in the United States. In some European nations parents are granted official work time without loss of pay in order to stay with their hospitalized young child; while in most instances, in the United States parents must take vacation time in order to remain in the hospital with their ill children. In many countries parents are not charged extra nor are more expensive rooms required when they stay overnight. In Great Britain plans for new hospitals must include adequate spatial provisions for parents to stay with their children on pediatric services. The authors hope that this special journal issue will contribute toward accelerating the rate of progress in this country over the next decade.

440. Shore, M. F., & Goldston, S. E. Mental health aspects of pediatric care: Historical view and current status. In P. R. Magrab (Ed.), Psychological management of pediatric problems. Volume I. Early life conditions and chronic diseases. Baltimore: University Park Press, 1978, 15-31.

Medical care in the United States currently is undergoing a major reevaluation in anticipation of a national health insurance program. As part of that evaluation, the components of high-quality comprehensive medical care are being redefined and described in the light of current knowledge. One result has been a rising interest in the mental health elements that should be included in any health service. The present concern about the mental health aspects of pediatric care can be seen as an outgrowth of three historical forces: the humanist tradition, the increased understanding of the close interweaving of biological and psychological elements, and the growing emphasis on preventing psychological dysfunctions in adult life. This chapter presents an overview of the field rather than an exhaustive review of the literature.

441. Shufer, S. Teaching via the play-discussion group. American Journal of Nursing, 1977, 77, 1960-1962.

A variety of methods are commonly used to help children cope with the events they will encounter during a hospital stay--prehospitalization tours and parties, introductory booklets, puppet shows, play with dolls and equipment, film strips, drawing, discussions, and demonstrations. This article discusses the play-discussion group as another way of reaching children. Although the merits of this type of activity on a pediatric unit in no way supercedes tours, booklets, individual preoperative preparation, or on-the-spot discussion of tests and procedures, it is a valuable supplemnt to all of these and has, in addition, merit as a teaching tool.

442. Sides, J. P. Emotional responses of children to physical illness and hospitalization (Doctoral dissertation, Auburn University, 1977). Dissertation Abstracts International, 1977, 38(2-B), 917.

Children hospitalized for physical illness were evaluated with regard to their behavior prior to, during, and after hospitalization by use of the Missouri Children's Behavior Checklist, the Missouri Children's Picture Series, selected Stanford-Binet subtests, Behavior Ratings Scales, the State-Trait Anxiety Inventory for Children, and a Posthospitalization Behavior Questionnaire. Idiographic data were also obtained. The children's mothers' anxiety levels were assessed with the State-Trait Anxiety Inventory. The number of subjects assessed on each variable ranged from 73 to 190. Multiple regression analyses identified variables contributing significantly to the prediction of posthospitalization behavior two weeks after discharge as consisting primarily of the child's behavioral response to medical treatment during hospitalization, the adequacy of the child's adjustment prior to hospitalization, idiographic variables, especially age, and the mother's anxiety level during her child's hospitalization. The results are interpreted as indicating that substantial numbers of children are emotionally upset by physical illness and hospitalization. Support is provided for the validity and utility of the instruments utilized in this study. The applicability of these results is discussed and specific research needs are identified.

443. Siegel, L. J. Reduction of anxiety in children facing hospitalization and surgery by use of filmed modeling (Doctoral dissertation, Case Western Reserve Univerity, 1975). Dissertation Abstracts International, 1975, 36 (6-B), 3071-3072.

The purpose of this study was to investigate the efficacy of filmed modeling, based on social learning theory, in reducing the emotional reactions of children hospitalized for surgery. Subjects were 60 children between the ages of four and twelve years old who were admitted to the hospital for the first time to undergo surgery for hernias, urinary-genital tract problems, or tonsillectomies. Statistical analysis of the data revealed a significant reduction in preoperative and postoperative anxiety for the subjects who viewed the hospital film. The state measures of anxiety consistently reflected differences between the two groups with the Experimental subjects showing lower sweat gland activity, fewer self-reported medical fears, and fewer anxiety related behaviors than the Control subjects. Measures of trait anxiety did not demonstrate a significant effect of the treatment conditions. Parents also reported a significant increase in the frequency and degree of behavior problems from the pre- to posthospitalization period for children in the Control group.

444. Siegel, L. J. Preparation of children for hospitalization: A selected review of the research literature. Journal of Pediatric Psychology, 1976, 1(4), 26-30.

An overview of the empirical literature on the preparation of children for hospitalization and surgery reveals a number of methodolgical inadequacies which subject the data to multiple interpretations. These investigations often lack appropriate control groups, do not control for relevant variables, and attempt to assess the child's emotional response to hospitalization without demonstrating the reliability of the measures used. As a result, the efficacy of a number of procedures presumed to facilitate the child's adjustment to the hospital experience remains to be clearly demonstrated.

445. Simonds, J. F. Psychiatric consultations for 112 pediatric patients. Southern Medical Journal, 1977, 70(8), 980-984.

The investigator studied 112 consecutive consultations, categorizing the presenting psychiatric problems, mental status, psychiatric diagnoses, final physical diagnoses, and psychiatric recommendations. The 112 patients represented 3.4% of all pediatric patients in the same age range admitted to the hospital. Girls comprised 59% of the sample studied. The most common presenting problems were unexplained physical symptoms, while the most frequent physical diagnoses were seizure disorder and diabetes. Psychiatric diagnoses were made for 82% of the patients seen; the most common diagnosis was "reactive" disorder. Specific recommendations for either inpatient or outpatient psychiatric care were made for 42 patients, of whom 23 were known to have followed through with the recommendations. However, most recommendations involved techniques that could be applied by the primary care physician, e.g., advice to parents, counseling the child, liaison with schools, direction of hospital staff.

446. Skellern, J. The self concept of children and adolescents and the effects of physical disability. Australasian Nurses Journal, 1979, 8(6), 36-38.

Self-concept refers to the ideas one has of oneself. It includes how one conceives the abstract parts of the self such as one's personality, value and identity. It also includes one's body image, the three dimensional view a person has of himself. This paper describes some of the cognitive and affective aspects of the development of self-concept considered sequentially, from infancy to adolescence, and discusses how it can be affected by bodily illness.

447. Smith, E. C., Liviskie, S. L., Nelson, K. A., & McNemar, A. Reestablishing a child's body image. American Journal of Nursing, 1977, 77(3), 445-447.

When a child suffers a disfiguring injury he responds as though his whole body has been hurt. With time and care, he is able to distinguish the injured part from the noninjured and eventually to incorporate that injury into how he sees himself. Observations of three children during their recovery periods led the authors to differentiate four stages they went through: (1) In the Global stage, the child does not distinguish one body part from another in either function, sensation, or appearance; (2) In the stage of Differentiation, the child discriminates changed body part from unchanged through sensation, function and appearance; (3) The stage of Articulation is characterized by testing and mastery of his sensorimotor skills with himself and others as well as his coordinating these experiences with his understanding of what has been done; and (4) At the point of Hierarchic integration, the child views his body as a whole and resumes his normal life.

448. Smith, J. C. Spending time with the hospitalized child. MCN: American Journal of Maternal Child Nursing, 1976, 1(3), 164.

This study examined whether nurses spend less time and/or make fewer contacts with hospitalized children when their parents are present. Results indicate that while the majority of nurses did not avoid seeing hospitalized children when their parents were with them, the majority of contacts were intended expressly for carrying out nursing procedures, not for interacting socially. Perhaps the most disturbing finding of this study is the fact that nurses spend an extremely brief time with a child during any given encounter, averaging less than a minute and a half. The author concludes that every nurse who cares for hospitalized children needs to reconsider what nursing care such youngsters require.

449. Smitherman, C. H. Parents of hospitalized children have needs, too. American Journal of Nursing, 1979, 79(8), 1423-1424.

Stress and anxiety of the hospitalized child often are related to the stress and anxiety that parents exhibit. This article outlines the following points about the needs of parents and ways of dealing with them: (1) parents need to see that their child is receiving competent physical care; (2) they need to understand the medical condition and treatment of their child; (3) they need to feel important to their children and capable as parents; (4) they need a chance to discuss their feelings about their child's hospitalization; and (5) parents may need to learn more about being honest with their children.

450. Snell, B., & Mclellan, C. Whetting hospitalized preschoolers' appetites. American Journal of Nursing, 1976, 76(3), 413-415.

Enticing hospitalized preschoolers to eat nutritionally sound meals is a chronic problem. Between the ages of 18 and 36 months, a toddler expresses two distinct phenomena: psychological negativism and physiological anorexia. The toddler simply says "No" in the majority of situations, including eating. Physiological anorexia results from a decrease in growth rate and weight gain in the second year. Once a child enters the hospital, anorexia may stem from his loss of autonomy, normal egocentric thought processes, and the effects of hospitalization. This article examines the problems of the hospitalized preschooler who will not eat, and suggestions for improving this situation are made.

451. Spenner, D. A preschool child copes with hospitalization. Maternal-Child Nursing Journal, 1974, 3(1), 41-48.

Hospitalization robs a child of his familiar surroundings and imposes upon him a new environment along with a new set of demands. The child does not choose to be hospitalized, yet he can do nothing to change the situation. He is often forced into a state of increased dependency and made to feel small, powerless, and insecure. He is subjected to numerous threats to body integrity, such as injections, surgery, and/or diagnostic procedures. This is a stressful experience for a child each time he is hospitalized, no matter how often he has been hospitalized in the past or how short the duration of his stay. This paper describes how one five-year-old boy coped with the stress of hospitalization, and his response to the attempts of a nurse to support his efforts toward mastery.

452. Spitz, R. A. Hospitalism: A follow-up report. In L. J. Stone, H. T. Smith, and L. B. Murphy (Eds.), The competent infant: Research and commentary. New York: Basic Books, Inc., 1973, 786-788.

This study offers a follow-up report to an original study also reported in this same edited text (Spitz, 1973). Of the original children studied at Foundling Home two years prior, 21 were still at the institution. The youngest was two years of age, the oldest four years and one month. Follow-up physical and psychological data indicated that the mental development of these 21 children was extraordinarily retarded, compared to that of normal children between the ages of two and four, who move, climb, and babble all day long, and who conform to or struggle against the educational demands of the environment. This retardation, which amounts to a deterioration, is borne out by the weights and heights of these children, as well as by their pictures.

453. Spitz, R. A. Hospitalism: An inquiry into the genesis of psychiatric conditions in early childhood. In L. J. Stone, H. T. Smith, and L. B. Murphy (Eds.), The competent infant: Research and commentary. New York: Basic Books, Inc., 1973, 775-786.

This study is especially concerned with the effect of continuous institutional care of infants under one year of age, for reasons other than sickness. The model of such institutions is the foundling home. A long-term study of 164 children confined to two institutions in different countries of the Western hemisphere was undertaken. A basis of comparison was established by investigating non-institutionalized children of the same age group in their parents' homes in both countries. In each case an anamnesis was made which whenever possible included data on the child's mother; and in each case the Hetzer-Wolf baby tests were administered. For the purpose of orientation the author established the average of the Developmental Quotients for the first third of the first year of life for each of the environments investigated and contrasted these averages with those for the last third of the first year. For children from professional homes in a large city, the Developmental Quotient (DQ), high from the start, remains high in the course of development. Children from an isolated fishing village show much lower DQ in the first four months and remain at a lower level than that of the previous category. In the third category, children handicapped from birth by the circumstances of their origin show DQ even somewhat lower than that of the village babaies; in the course of their development they gain slightly. In the fourth category, "Foundling Home," the children are of an unselected urban (Latin) background. Their DQ on admission is below that of the best category but much higher than that of the other two. The picture changes completely by the end of the first year, when their Developmental Quotient sinks to an astonishingly low level.

454. Spivack, M. Helping a child in the hospital: A father's story. Journal of the Association for the Care of Children in Hospitals, 1979, 7(3), 11-13.

This article describes the experiences of a family whose two-year-old child went into the hospital. The father and the hospitalized child's three-year-old brother made a tape with songs and stories to bring to the younger boy in order to give him some sounds of home when they could not be with him. The reactions of the sick child are described, and the feelings of the family discussed.

455. Stacey, M. Conclusions of the case-study sample. In M. Stacey (Ed.), Hospitals, children and their families: The report of a pilot study. London: Routledge & Kegan Paul, Ltd., 1970, 127-148.

This chapter examines the data gathered on a sample of children who entered one of two hospitals for tonsillectomy and adenoidectomy, to see whether there are hypotheses derivable from a psycho-sociological examination of the data which did not emerge from separate psychiatric and sociological investigations. Although this was a small pilot study and the data must be considered with caution, some substantive findings emerged. Examination of the psycho-social data taken together revealed more about the normals, those who survived hospital without being labelled as maladjusted, disturbed or behaving atypically in the ward, than it did about the latter categories. The study shows at least some of the characteristics of those who survive as normal. These characteristics are described and discussed.

456. Stacey, M. Introduction. In M. Stacey (Ed.), Hospitals, children and their families: The report of a pilot study. London: Routledge & Kegan Paul, Ltd., 1970, 1-13.

This introductory chapter describes research undertaken by the School of Social Studies, University College, Swansea, Wales, in 1964. The aim of the research was to establish certain facts and relationships about children in hospital which were: (a) social; (b) psychiatric; and (c) resulted from a combination of both. The social research aimed: (1) to relate the socio-economic status and family structure of child in-patients to the visiting they receive; (2) to establish the inhibitors, apart from hospital regulations, to living in or to visiting by the mother, father or mother substitute; and (3) to establish the social relations of the child in the ward, his relationship during in-patient stay with his parents and hospital staff. The psychiatric research aimed to show whether there is a relationship between emotional disturbance and separation from the mother in the hospital situation and to investigate other variables related to children in hospital. The aim in reporting the research throughout the book is to show the implications of the findings for the administration of the hospital service.

457. Stacey, M. The practical implications of our conclusions. In D. Hall and M. Stacey (Eds.), Beyond separation: Further studies of children in hospital. London: Routledge & Kegan Paul, Ltd., 1979, 179-216.

This chapter presents an overview of the research on children in hospital which is reported and discussed in this volume. The concern is with child patients rather than simply with pediatric patients. The most important practical implication of this book and the work it reports is that it asks that the therapy of children should be redefined to include the sociological and psychological aspects. The findings therefore have implications of a profound kind for those who work with sick children, who are concerned with policy-making or who are involved in the education of health-care professionals. Several practical recommendations are made: the first is a program of education and training designed to encourage the re-thinking which is necessary for changes to be made in the care of children in hospital; the second relates to organizational changes; and the third concerns suggestions for further research.

458. Stacey, M. Practical recommendations. In M. Stacey (Ed.), Hospitals, children and their families: The report of a pilot study. London: Routledge & Kegan Paul, Ltd., 1970, 149-159.

This chapter summarizes the findings of a study undertaken on a sample of children who entered one of two hospitals for tonsillectomy and adenoidectomy. The implications of the data for hospital practice is discussed.

459. Stanford, G. Now is the time: The professionalization of child life workers. Journal of the Association for the Care of Children in Hospitals, 1980, 8(3), 55-59.

A profession is like a child. It, too, changes and develops over the years, both maturing and responding to changing conditions. Like a child's development, the growth of a profession progresses in spurts and reaches plateaus: sometimes growing rapidly, at other times more slowly; sometimes facing crucial issues, other times consolidating previous changes. And like the development of a child, the growth of a profession can be influenced somewhat, but cannot be completely controlled. This article explores the developmental stages of the child life profession, and discusses how to help a profession which is in its adolescence get through the storms and struggles into maturity. To have "come of age," a profession must possess a number of attributes, many of which the child life profession has already taken on. Three key elements, however, have been lacking in this profession: (1) a clearly defined role; (2) clearly defined qualifications; and (3) control over entry into the profession. Suggestions are offered as to how these elements can be acquired to enable the child life profession to grow into professional adulthood.

460. Steele, S. General ideas in relation to long-term illness in childhood. In S. Steele (Ed.), Nursing care of the child with long-term illness. New York: Appleton-Century-Crofts, 1971, 97-132.

The child with a long-term illness can be a real challenge to nurses, as well as other medical personnel and to his family. The child develops some unique qualities which are formulated as a result of living with an illness. In planning nursing care, the student should keep in mind that these factors will influence the overall plan of care. Too frequently nurses have a tendency to respond only to immediate pressures rather than planning care to incorporate expected behaviors. This chapter discusses some of these expected behaviors for consideration and utilization in planning and executing patient care.

461. Stephens, K. S. A toddler's separation anxiety. American Journal of Nursing, 1973, 73(9), 1553-1555.

This article describes the hospitalization of a young child for a unilateral cleft lip operation. Immediately after her mother left, Rose sat down on the playroom floor and wet her pants. When a nurse attempted to remove her to a room to change her, she cried and screamed and kicked the nurse. She may have interpreted the loss of her mother as punishment for previous wrong-doing and thus guilt was added to grief, and the two-year-old was in total emotional turmoil. Abandoned in a strange place by the one person whom she loved, she felt unwanted, unimportant and deserted. An hour after her mother left, Rose had already moved into despair. When the mother returned, the child responded by rejecting her. Only after some hours was the mother able to stimulate her to respond favorably.

462. Stocking, M., Rothney, W., Grosser, G., & Goodwin, R. Psychopathology in the pediatric hospital: Implications for the pediatrician. Psychiatry in Medicine, 1970, 1(4), 329-338.

A study of the incidence and range of psychopathology in a random sample of admissions to a pediatric hospital revealed: (a) an unexpectedly high incidence of children manifesting psychopathology or difficulties in emotional adaptation considered by the child psychiatrist to warrent psychiatric consultation (63.7 percent); (b) the pediatric staff requested consultation on nine of 51 of these children (17.6 percent) considered to manifest difficulties in emotional adaptation. Factors including the acuteness of medical illness, its treatability, the age of the child, and the nature of the emotional disorder were found to be related to the pediatrician's failure to recognize the need for consultation. The usefulness of random screening procedures is considered as a teaching device to alert pediatricians to the existence of psychopathology which they otherwise might not recognize.

463. Stocking, M., Rothney, W., Grosser, G., & Goodwin, R. Psychopathology in the pediatric hospital--implications for community health. American Journal of Public Health, 1972, 62(4), 551-556.

With the hope of contributing knowledge to a neglected area the authors undertook a study designed: (1) to find the incidence of psychopathology in children admitted to a pediatric hospital; (2) to delineate how often such psychopathology is not recognized by the pediatric staff; and (3) to find the frequency with which children are hospitalized unnecessarily. A random sample of every twentieth child admitted to a pediatric hospital over a ten-month period was selected for study. The parent (with one exception, the mother) of each child was interviewed by a child psychiatrist within the first 48 hours of the child's admission to the hospital. The following results are reported: (1) Of the children in the sample 63.7% were in need of psychiatric consultation; (2) The pediatric ward staff requested psychiatric consultation on only 11.3% of the sample; (3) Child psychiatrist and pediatrician agreed that approximately 70% of the children clearly needed hospitalization. The child psychiatrist felt that for 30% it was not necessary and was disadvantageous. The pediatrician regarded admission as not essential, but advantageous, for approximately 17% of the sample, and as clearly neither needed nor advantageous for 12.5% of the children studied; (4) In the group of children for whom hospitalization was judged unnecessary, the incidence of psychopathology was particularly great. Twenty-four of the twenty-seven children were independently judged to show signs of emotional disturbance. This study suggests that the pediatric hospital is already serving as a mental health resource to a large number of children, without any well-planned program to meet their needs. The hospital's usefulness as a resource is currently limited by the fact that too often hospitalization is used by the parent, and the doctor as well, to deny the child's emotional difficulty, rather than to delineate the child's emotional needs to help the child and his parents to achieve a realistic psychological adaptation.

464. Streissguth, A. P., & Streissguth, D. M. Planning for the psychological needs of a young child in a double spica cast. Clinical Pediatrics, 1978, 17(3), 277-283.

The two phases of treatment of the young child in a full spica cast stimulate two different psychological needs on the part of the young patient. Understanding them should enable parents to cope more effectively. These needs include: (1) While in the cast, the child experiences strong needs to maintain autonomy and mobility. Parents can help by maintaining as normal as possible social and academic activities; (2) After the cast is removed the child may feel vulnerable and helpless and be temporarily more dependent than the parents are likely to be prepared for. It is important that the child be allowed to progress at his own pace without being made to feel guilty about not recovering more rapidly.

465. Sullivan, K. Hospital play sessions. Maternal-Child Nursing Journal, 1972, 1(2), 187-192.

This article describes the play sessions of a five and one-half year old girl who experienced multiple hospitalizations for surgical correction of a lumbo-sacral myelomeningocele, hydrocephalus, shunt revisions, bilateral congenital dislocated hips, and other orthopedic problems. This child differed from other children her age most remarkably in the area of limited mobility and the absence of bladder control. One of the major themes portrayed in play sessions was her concern about body integrity, especially the inability to control her bladder, which resulted in a constant state of urinary incontinence, and which necessitated the use of diapers as a part of her apparel.

466. Suran, B. G., & Hatcher, R. P. The psychological treatment of hospitalized children with failure-to-thrive. Pediatric Nursing, 1975, 1(5), 10-17.

This article attempts to redefine the failure-to-thrive syndrome in children who present without specific organic symptoms other than inability to maintain adequate weight-gain. Failure-to-thrive is seen as a psychological disturbance secondary to poor psychosocial adaptation, having its origin in a number of factors including environmental deprivation, a disturbed family system, or an inherent inability to assimilate normal experiences. A specific, psychosocial stimulation program for the hospitalized child is suggested with the intent of helping the child reorganize mental-emotional structures.

467. Suran, B. G., & Lavigne, J. V. Rights of children in pediatric settings: A survey of attitudes. Pediatrics, 1977, 60(5), 715-720.

This study compares the attitudes of parents and health care professionals toward the bill of rights for children in pediatric settings of the National Association of Children's Hospitals and Related Institutions (NACHRI) and a locally developed ombudsman committee bill of rights. Parents (N = 64), attending physicians (N = 33), resident physicians (N = 17), nurses (N = 27), nonmedical professionals (N = 35), administrators (N = 18), and clerical workers (N = 17) were surveyed. Each person rated statements derived from the bills from "strongly agree" to "strongly disagree." Analyses of variance indicated a high level of agreement overall for both bills by all groups; however, the local bill was significantly preferred. There were significant differences in agreement between the groups for the local bill and the two bills combined (an overall measure of attitudes about children's rights in pediatric settings). Attending physicians tended to agree significantly less than other groups. Of the 32 individual items, attending or resident physicians were significantly lower in agreement than most other groups on 11 items, and nurses were lowest on one other. Disagreement was strongest on items concerning abortion or contraception, the child's right to privacy, the right to consent to care, and the right to have an immediate response from the physician in understandable language.

468. Swanson, V. M. Pediatric schoolroom: An oasis of normalcy. Journal of the Association for the Care of Children in Hospitals, 1979, 7(3), 17-19.

This article describes a school program at the Delaware Division Hospital of the Wilmington Medical Center which is structured to meet the needs of both long- and short-term patients from kindergarten through 12th grade. The purpose of this pediatric school program is threefold: (1) to provide constructive activity, academic involvement, and peer association for all hospitalized students; (2) to provide the opportuntity for the long-term patient to keep up with the specific subject matter from the home school; and (3) to provide an oasis of normalcy within unfamiliar and often threatening surroundings.

469. Swanson, V. M. The school-age traction patient: Toward better behavior patterns. Journal of the Association for the Care of Children in Hospitals, 1980, 9(1), 12-14.

A myriad of medical problems are more serious, more traumatic, and more life threatening than the fractured femur, but few are more confining, more uncomfortable, and more frustrating than being immobilized when the remainder of the body is apparently reasonably healthy. Placing the pediatric pateint in the appropriate orthopedic rigging triggers off a succession of dilemmas with which the child must deal. Feelings he displays produce actions with which staff and family must cope. Thus, identifying both feelings and progressive stages of activity that the child in traction experiences can be helpful to the hospital staff upon whom demands are continuously made by this "less ill than other" child and to the family who will interact for a lengthy period of time with this incapacitated child.

470. Sweeney, L., & Zingher, G. Hospitalization enhances creativity. Journal of the Association for the Care of Children in Hospitals, 1979, 7(3), 14-16.

It seems that the event of illness and hospitalization can be an extraordinary life experience, which may accentuate the inner need to create. This heightened creative drive goes beyond the normal, innovative play experience which the healthy child initiates joyfully at all stages of his or her development. The nature of the hospitalization experience, imposing bodily hurt, and physical and psychological separation from family and normal life, may indeed heighten a child's need to struggle for a sense of separate, individual selfhood. This article discusses creativity in the hospitalized child, and presents the case of a 14-year-old boy hospitalized periodically for treatment of Hodgkin's disease as illustration.

471. Taylor, F. L. Educational preparation for surgery: An examination of physical and behavioral parameters post-operatively (Doctoral dissertation, Case Western Reserve University, 1977). Dissertation Abstracts International, 1978, 38(11-A), 6416.

The purpose of the present study was to determine the effect of systematic educational pre-operative instruction on selected physical and behavioral findings post-operatively. The study demonstrated significant differences in amount of post-operative vomiting and in the amount of pain medication given post-operatively between the control and the experimental groups. There were also significant differences on these criterion due to age regardless of placement in the experimental or control groups. There were also significant differences found in the rates of respiration throughout the hospitalization. These differences were due to age rather than to group placement. Certain aspects of the child's behavior were also affected by surgery. Children in the experimental group showed less fear of strangers, fewer temper tantrums, and less worry about trips to the doctor's office than did those children in the control group.

472. Tekely, K., & Dittermore, I. Regressive behavior in a hospitalized preschool child. Maternal-Child Nursing Journal, 1978, 7(3), 185-190.

This article presents the case study of a four-year-old child who had experienced repeated, traumatic and prolonged hospitalizations because of chronic illness. The child dealt with hospitalization and illness by regression to earlier levels of psychosocial development in play and object relationships. To deny separation anxiety she avoided play with a separation theme and actively avoided conversations or reference to her natural mother. Instead, she used behavior which tended to promote a more symbiotic type of relationship. The majority of her behaviors evidenced ambivalence to mother, reminiscent of the anal sadistic stage. The torture aspect of anal behavior was particularly apparent. The child concentrated on working through the anxiety brought about by separation from home, her illness and the trauma of hospitalization.

473. Terry, G. A five year old boy's aggressive and compensatory behavior in response to immobilization. Maternal-Child Nursing Journal, 1979, 8(1), 29-38.

This article presents the case study of a five-year-old boy (Jamie) hospitalized for osteomyelitis. The author reviews the behavior of this minor, pointing out that Jamie's two major coping strategies, aggressive behaviors and compensatory ways of achieving motility, were appropriate and typical for his age. At times, Jamie's instinctual impulses, especially his aggressive impulse, were so powerful that his ego control diminished and allowed his aggressive feelings to dominate. Occasionally, he expressed his aggression in primitive forms. This behavior was evident when he used his teeth to bite after he had used a puppet for the same purpose. Jamie dealt with his strong drive for motility in a less primitive way. In fact, he drew upon his cognitive abilities to find such alternate ways of achieving motion as thinking of reasons to get up in the cart or initiating play which involved movement of objects. Jamie's use of aggressive behavior and compensatory ways of achieving motility appeared to increase as the period of motility restriction continued. When he was finally allowed to walk without restriction, Jamie no longer needed to find compensatory ways of achieving motility. But his use of aggressive behavior persisted until he was discharged home. His use of these two coping mechanisms enabled him to go through his twenty day hospital experience without being overwhelmed.

474. Tesler, M., & Hardgrove, C. Cardiac catheterization: Preparing the child. American Journal of Nursing, 1973, 73(1), 80-82.

This article describes the preparation of children for cardiac catheterization the day before the procedure and in the presence of a parent. Preparation is seen as a two stage affair: precatheterization and postcatheterization. In the precatheterization visit, the concentration is on describing the known facts about the procedure. What the child will experience and what he can do to help himself is emphasized. During the postcatheterization interview, the child is allowed the triumph and satisfaction of reporting his special feelings about the experience and his pride in having survived. This mastery can boost self-esteem, making the experience a step rather than a block in his development. It also helps separate reality from fantasy--what happened from what he thought happened. At no point is the seriousness of the medical implications of cardiac catheterization minimized, but an attempt is made to communicate to the child that he is not going through the experience alone.

475. Thompson, R. H., & Stanford, G. Coping with resistance to child life programming. Journal of the Association for the Care of Children in Hospitals, 1978, 7(4), 12-18.

As more is understood about the emotional effects of hospitalization on young people, hospitals are increasingly making deliberate attempts to reduce the stress of a hospital stay on young patients and their parents. These changes--which may range from new policies governing parent visitation to the development of comprehensive play programs and pre-admission orientation tours--are often referred to as "child life programming." Usually trained child life workers are responsible for planning and implementing child life interventions. Although other professionals in the hospital can usually be counted on to lend support to changes made to ameliorate the psychological effects of hospitalization, it is virtually inevitable that there will be some opposition from other groups within the hospital. This article discusses opposition which can emerge because the role and function of the child life worker may parallel or conflict with those of another group within the hospital system--whether it be administration, medical staff, nursing staff, mental health services, volunteer services, or occupational therapy.

476. Tiedt, E. The adolescent in the hospital: An identity-resolution approach. Nursing Forum, 1972, 11(2), 121-140.

Adolescents face, according to Erikson, an identity search composed of seven interrelated dimensions, presenting them with constant challenges and tasks to arrive at their own identity. Hospitalization imposes on these dimensions an unfamiliar setting which leads to anxiety; demands for extra attention, explanations, and support in limit-setting; separation from family, peers, and school. It provokes dependency, regression, and insecurity that may be manifested by temper outbursts, crying, the need for dependence; and it increases concern about body-concept and sexuality aroused by the illness, exposure, and loss of privacy. Effective nursing intervention techniques can help the adolescent use appropriate coping measures in continuing his identity resolution while faced with the added stress of hospitalization. The way in which the adolescent is cared for, physically and mentally, and the attention and understanding he receives, will influence (positively or negatively) his own ideology or philosophy of life. Nursing personnel affect this and should be aware of this influence. Hospitalization for the adolescent can become a positive, identity-developing experience when nursing interventions are based on an understanding of the adolescent and the tasks involved in his identity search.

477. Tisza, V. B., Hurwitz, I., & Angoff, K. The use of a play program by hospitalized children. Journal of the American Academy of Child Psychiatry, 1970, 9, 515-531.

A research project was designed to study the play activity of hospitalized children in the playroom of a hospital for children. The project was restricted to the description and analysis of observational data during the first three days in the playroom, and is a combined cross-sectional and longitudinal study--a developmental study within a brief time span. Children belonging to three age groups were observed: three- to four-year-olds, four- to six-year-olds, and six- to eight-year olds. The focus was on the description of the children's affective responses and a wide range of other behavioral manifestations. In this paper only the first and third age groups are discussed in detail; the reactions of the transitional middle group are briefly mentioned. The study demonstrated the importance of the continuity of supportive relationships for young hospitalized children. If relationships are offered, not even the three- to four-year olds experience the absence of the parent as so profound a loss, because of the relative stability of the introjected image of the parent. However, the study also points out that the external and internal threats inherent in the hospital experience create so much anxiety that, at least during the first three days in the playroom, children of the age groups studied are largely unable to master the situation through dramatic play.

During the initial period of hospitalization they either regress or struggle against regression, with resultant primitivization or even absence of play activity.

478. Toker, E. Psychiatric aspects of cardiac surgery in a child. Journal of the American Academy of Child Psychiatry, 1971, 10(1), 156-186.

Some of the literature on the significance of the heart in mythology and folklore has been reviewed in addition to literature on the psychiatric aspects of heart surgery. Furthermore, the case of a seven-year-old Puerto Rican girl was presented and her problems prior to and following heart surgery were reviewed. Finally, five psychotherapy sessions with this patient and nine of her H-T-P drawings were included and the salient features discussed.

479. Tonkin, P. Parent care for the low risk and terminally ill child. Dimensions in Health Service, 1979, 56(5), 42-43.

This article describes the development of a care by parent unit at Children's Hospital in Vancouver. It is a separate geographic unit attached to an acute surgical ward, designed to be as similar to the home environment as possible. There is a brightly colored lounge with appropriate furniture, color television and a snack bar with refrigerator and stove. The children are cared for mainly by their parents with the guidance and assistance of the nursing staff, who are dressed in practical street clothes. Parents of the children admitted to the care by parent unit are overwhelmingly in favor of taking an active role in their child's hospitalization. This unit provides parents with this opportunity. Realizing that hospitalization can have major emotional consequences for a child, parents and health care professionals benefit greatly from working and sharing together in a care by parent unit, and can thereby minimize the trauma often associated with hospitalization.

480. Treloar, D. M. Ready, set--no: Something is missing from pediatric pre-op preparation. MCN: American Journal of Maternal Child Nursing, 1978, 3(1), 50-51.

Hospitalization itself is traumatic enough for most youngsters, fraught with painful procedures, strange manipulations, and age- and development-specific stresses. Surgery or a major diagnostic procedure compounds all these problems, for the extent to which children can fantasize about the unknown is overwhelming. It is suggested that one way the nurse can help children master these fears is by thorough, thoughtful preparation and education. A checklist which ensures the child's thorough preparation for the strange events he will encounter is presented.

481. Tsignounis, S. A., Jr. The relationship between parent-child perceptions of hospitalization and the child's subsequent psychological response (Doctoral dissertation, California School of Professional Psychology, 1977). Dissertation Abstracts International, 1978, 38 (8-B), 3915.

The intent of the study was to examine the relationships between parent-child perceptions of hospitalization when the child was pending minor surgery, and the child's subsequent psychological response and post-hospital perceptions. Twenty-six families who had a child pending hospitalization for minor surgery were interviewed pre- and post-hospitalization to assess perception variables, background variables, and psychological response variables. The findings of this study suggest that perception variables are good predictors of the child's post-hospital psychological response. These perception variables include the child's perceptions of self-anxiety, his perceptions of the severity of the surgery, his perceptions of his parents' anxiety, and his satisfaction with the information he has received regarding the hospitalization. The parents' perceptions include their perceptions of their own anxiety, their perceptions of their child's adjustment, and their satisfaction with the information received regarding the hospitalization. Important background variables include the child's participation in a hospital preparation program, and the frequency of the child's previous hospitalizations. Another significant finding was the fact that the child manifested more behavior problems prior to hospitalization than after hospitalization. This suggests that physicians and nurses need to be aware that imparting too much information too early may cause an increase in behavior problems prior to hospitalization. No significant relationship was found between any variable and the child's post-hospital perceptions. No significant relationship was found between the parents' perceptions of hospitalization and the child's perceptions of hospitalization. No sex differences were found.

482. Tureman, C. A., & Johnson, P. A. Observing and recording behaviors of hospitalized children. Journal of the Association for the Care of Children in Hospitals, 1977, 6(1), 17-22.

Child Life workers and teachers in the hospital setting have unusual opportunities to contribute valuable data to the medical assessment team. These staff members usually have had training in child development and education; thus, they are competent observers of child behavior. Their close interaction with the hospitalized child, be it in caretaking, recreational or educational activities, presents a unique perspective in a nonthreatening situation. Observation and recording of behavior could provide needed information that would assist the medical team in developing a regimen of adequate care. It is hoped that this article will be helpful for nurses, social workers and other related disciplines in the hospital setting, as well as Child Life workers as a group.

483. Uzark, K. A child's cardiac catheterization: Avoiding the potential risks. MCN: American Journal of Maternal Child Nursing, 1978, 3(3), 158-161.

Cardiac catheterization is usually done before a child with a heart defect reaches school age. The separation from parents which is often required during his hospitalization for the procedure is especially traumatic for children at this age. Parents and staff are two critical determinants of the child's reaction. If the child can learn from his experiences and come to trust health care professionals and from them, people in general, his hospitalization for cardiac catheterization will be a source of psychological benefit. The nursing staff's awareness of the factors discussed in this article can contribute in many ways to making the experience a very positive one for the child and his family, the family can be helped to cope with the hospitalization, the accuracy and safety of the catheterization procedure can be ensured, and, finally, an invaluable attitude of co-operation and trust can be fostered in the child.

484. van den Berg, J. H. Dubious maternal affection. Pittsburgh: Duquesne University Press, 1972.

This book suggests that too much affection towards our children, especially of the wrong type, is worse than not enough affection. The author takes as his point of departure the views concerning hospitalism--the lack of adequate psychological care provided infants in hospitals and foundling homes--as they were originally formulated in the years immediately following World War II. He shows how the results were interpreted in a way that went beyond the evidence, and in a direction that fit therapists' biases, and how the popularization of Freudian views helped sustain the exaggeration of the interpretation. The author also maintains that the effect on adulthood of early childhood traumas has been unduly exaggerated.

485. van der Schyff, G. The role of parents during their child's hospitalization. Australasian Nurses Journal, 1979, 8(11), 57-58, 61.

A continuing relationship with the parents is necessary for the emotional well-being of the hospitalized child. Satisfactory parent participation in the care of the child in hospital depends upon the definition, and acceptance, of the role of the parent in hospital. There are several factors which can impede or facilitate role function. The provision of cues by hospital staff to parents increases the adequacy of parents relating to their hospitalized child. Parents need to acquaint themselves with what their role should be. Inclusion of the parents in the care of their child in hospital has many advantages for staff, parents and child.

486. Van Krevelen, D. A. Hospitalism. Acta Paedopsychiatrica, 1970, 37(2), 45.

The concept of hospitalism, the origin of which is to be found in last century pediatrics, has come into fashion in today's child psychiatry, resulting in strong resistances in professional circles against referring young children to hospitals, children's homes and institutions. In this connection two measures have been proposed, viz. simultaneous admission of the young patient and his mother, and continuation of treatment on an out-patient basis, until the necessity of clinical treatment outweighs the disadvantages which placement outside the family environment is supposed to involve. Both alternatives encounter difficulties. To begin with, combined admission of mother and child is not only a burden for nurses and other staff members, it also implies a complication for the little patient himself. The mother's projection of her insufficiency feelings upon other adults who take over her role, adds to her existing uncertainty. As to the second measure, it is foredoomed to failure, because influences which aggravate the disease--psychical factors--go on prevailing. In both cases no advantage is taken of the therapeutic value of separation. It is the author's experience that children in hospital can better stand separation from their parents than the latter can bear their children's absence. Hence, he feels it would be preferable to speak of "hospitalism of parents."

487. Vardaro. J. A. R. Preadmission anxiety and mother-child relationships. Journal of the Association for the Care of Children in Hospitals, 1978, 7(2), 8-15.

The purpose of the study described in this article was to investigate if there is a relationship between anxiety in the preschool child and anxiety in the parent prior to hospitalization of the child for elective surgery. The specific hypothesis tested was: Anxiety in the parent prior to hospitalization of his or her preschool child for elective surgery will significantly correlate with the anxiety in his or her preschool child. The data in this study support the "emotional contagion hypothesis" set forth in the literature, which points out that a parent's emotional state may be transmitted to a young child. Implications of the results are discussed.

488. Vermilion, B. D., Ballantine, T. V., & Grosfeld, J. L. The effective use of the parent care unit for infants on the surgical service. Journal of Pediatric Surgery, 1979, 14(3), 321-324.

There is little information available concerning the management of pediatric surgical patients on a Parent Care Unit. Review of a six-year experience with 141 patients has demonstrated that pediatric surgical patients with special problems benefit from a period of care on such a unit. Patients ranged in age from five days to 12 years. Indications for admission included post-operative training, prolonged parent-child separation, preoperative hospitalization, post-operative recovery, and diagnostic work-up. Sixty-eight percent of the patients had congenital anomalies while 5% were admitted with infectious processes, 3% tumors, and 24% had miscellaneous disorders. The Parent Care Unit (PCU) provides a controlled and protected environment within the hospital setting in which the parents have an opportunity to overcome their fears of inadequacy and to develop expertise in the management of their children's disabilities and/or appliances. The emotional trauma experienced by the child is lessened on a PCU while quality of parent participation is enhanced by appropriate instruction techniques. The PCU costs only 70% the cost of a routine inpatient bed and, thus, appeals to advocates of cost containment and efficient utilization of hospital staff. By removing the child from the mainstream of the hospital, the risk of cross-infection between patients is reduced. The quality of subsequent home management is significantly enhanced by this experience that diminishes the psychological trauma associated with hospital discharge and home responsibility. This adjustment is of particular importance in instances of prolonged parent-child separation associated with complicated birth defects. The PCU is a useful adjunct in the surgical care of infants and its use and development should be encouraged and extended.

489. Visintainer, M. The effects of pre-admission psychological preparation on children's stress responses and adjustment during and following hospitalization for minor surgery. Nursing Research Report, 1977, 12(1), 3-5.

The psychological distress that children experience in the hospital is of major concern to all who work in pediatrics. Consequently, attempts to help children deal with the painful procedures, separation, surgery, and other stressful events have produced many changes and innovations on pediatric units. This article describes a series of investigations to try to understand psychological preparation and to study the effects that it had on children undergoing surgery. The author concludes that comprehensive psychological preparation and planned supportive care are complicated affairs which require a well articulated theoretical base and careful integration into ongoing care. Both nursing and medical staff have to be much better informed about the principles and techniques of psychological preparation if they are going to use them effectively. No single theoretical construct is sufficient as a basis for a program of preparation and supportive care.

490. Visintainer, M. A., & Wolfer, J. A. Psychological preparation for surgical pediatric patients: The effect on children's and parents' stress responses and adjustment. Pediatrics, 1975, 56(2), 187-202.

This clinical experiment tested variations of psychological preparation and supportive care designed to increase the adjustment of children (and their parents) hospitalized for elective surgery. Eighty-four children, aged three to 12, admitted for tonsillectomies were randomly assigned to one of three treatment conditions or to a control group: (1) a combination of systematic preparation, rehearsal, and supportive care conducted prior to each stressful procedure; (2) a single-session preparation conducted after admission; and (3) consistent supportive care given by one nurse at the same points as in the first condition, but including no systematic preparation or rehearsal. The children's hospital adjustment was measured by blind ratings of behavioral upset and cooperation during the blood test, medication injection, transport to surgery, induction, and postoperative fluid intake and by recovery room medications and pulse rates and time to first voiding. Post-hospital adjustment was assessed with Vernon _et al_.'s Post Hospital Behavior Inventory. Parent outcome measures included self-ratings for anxiety and satisfaction with information and care. As hypothesized, the results demonstrated that children who received condition one showed significantly less upset and more cooperation and their parents reported significantly greater satisfaction and less anxiety than did children or parents in the other groups. Younger children were significantly more upset and less cooperative than older children.

491. Waidley, E. Preparing children for radiology procedure. _Journal of the Association for the Care of Children in Hospitals_, 1977, _6_(1), 6-11.

In this article the author stresses the needs of children undergoing radiology procedures and the variables that will affect the success of any method of preparation. Important facts that should be used as guidelines when planning a radiology preparation program include: (1) Effective preparation must be timely, well-organized, complete, and factual; (2) Each child should be assessed prior to the preparation in order to determine his/her individual learning and developmental needs; (3) Parental involvement during preparation and/or during the procedure if allowed offers the child a trusting and reliable support system before and after the x-ray; (4) Adequate time must be alloted during the preparation for child's and parents' questions and answers, and after the procedure for verbalization and playing-out; and (5) Adults who work with children in unfamiliar and stressful situaiton must evaluate their own communication patterns and adapt them to the child's needs.

492. Wear, E. T. Separation anxiety reconsidered: Nursing implications. _Maternal-Child Nursing Journal_, 1974, _3_(1), 9-18.

The intent of this paper is (a) to present two reports that summarize the child's behavioral reactions to separation; (b) to offer two authors' opinions about the nature of the child's tie to his mother and the origin of separation anxiety; and (c) to discuss the meaning these have for nursing practice. Several nursing interventions aimed toward alleviating separation anxiety in the young hospitalized child are suggested: (a) provision of continuous, individualized care of the child by a limited number of nursing personnel; (b) measures to support the child in coping with his feelings; (c) nurturance of a sense of competency in the child; (d) provision of familair clothing, foods, etc.; and (e) provision of sights and sounds of the loved parents.

493. Weaver, L., & Schlegel, D. Planning a nutrition program for the hospital playroom. Journal of the Association for the Care of Children in Hospitals, 1976, 5(1), 20-22.

This article describes a program at Children's Hospital, Columbus, Ohio, where patients can learn about good nutrition in the hospital playroom. Members of the Dietary Department and the Patient Activity Department at the hospital have developed a weekly nutrition activity program for children on the surgical unit. Many types of lessons are taught in these programs, and all of them deal with good nutrition in a play therapy setting. Many of the nutrition activities involve food preparation. The project has increased the dietitians' knowledge of child development, and the activity therapist has learned a great deal about food composition and nutrition. Goals for the patients and program are described and discussed.

494. Webb, B. Trauma and tedium: An account of living-in on a children's ward. In A. Davis and G. Horobin (Eds.), Medical encounters: The experience of illness and treatment. London: Croom Helm, 1977, 175-190.

Documentation of the observable effects of hospitalization on young children has contributed to changes in British hospital and governmental policies with regard to the presence of the child's parents on the ward, e.g., unrestricted visiting, overnight stays in hospital and the importation of the mother into the hospital with the child. The effects on ward interactions of a mother's continual presence is of interest sociologically. It is a unique situation in the hospital, to have a patient's aide and representative present throughout all routine ward procedures, as both an observer and a participant. The pattern of staff-parent-child relations which emerges provides insights into the way knowledge is acquired and used by the participant-observer within the hierarchical structure of the hospital. This chapter presents the account of a mother who lived in hospital with her burned child.

495. Weiss, H. H., & Pizer, E. F. Hospitalizing the young: Is it for their own good? Mental Hygiene, 1970, 54(4), 498-502.

The authors question the advisability of hospitalization for children and adolescents, arguing that their admission for treatment may have long term deleterious effects on them. Among these are the stigma attached to hospitalization, the impact on self-concept, reduced opportunities for future self-determination and the possibility of diminished social competence. Juveniles should not be denied hospitalization for treatment when indicated, but this action should only be taken after careful deliberation of all the consequences.

496. Welch, C. The nurse's role in play. Nursing Care, 1977, 10(1), 14-15.

Children use play as a tool to express themselves, to experiment, and to learn about their environment. Play helps children cope with stress and anxiety, especially in a clinical setting. This article describes a therapeutic play program in effect at Philadelphia Children's Hospital which was insituted to promote a healthy attitude among patients toward their illnesses.

497. Wessell, M. L. Use of humor by an immobilized adolescent girl during hospitalization. Maternal-Child Nursing Journal, 1975, 4(1), 35-48.

Ann, the subject of the present study, was admitted to the hospital for the first time at fifteen years of age for treatment of scoliosis. From the first day that the nurse met Ann and throughout her extended hospitalization, it became obvious that humor held a unique place in her way of behaving and rising above this anxiety-provoking situation. During hospitalization, Ann found herself immobilized in a cast that restricted the patterns of behavior used in the past to relieve frustration and discharge aggression. Ann's manner of dealing with controllable anxiety was consistent throughout her hospitalization. It was characterized by her sense of humor. Her ready laughter and pleasant manner helped Ann make friends with many people in the hospital environment. Ann found an acceptable outlet for aggression in the subtle and indirect type of attack offered by aggressive humor. At times, for her own psychic economy, Ann withdrew her energy inward to struggle with her pain or powerful emotions, but always returned with her characteristic smile and sense of humor to relations with others.

498. Wheeler, W. E. Recollections of 40 years of hospitalization of children. Pediatric Research, 1972, 6(11), 840-842.

This article discusses the author's experiences with children in hospitals. The changes and developments of hospital care are described, and some of the problems experienced by him are discussed.

499. White, P. Hospital recreation helps adolescent patients. Canadian Nurse, 1972, 68(7), 34-35.

This article discusses a program at The Hospital for Sick Children in Toronto, where staff members work with adolescent patients to help them express their emotions in ways that are positive. The facilities include a large complex of rooms furnished with pool and ping pong tables, color television, stereo, refrigerator, and stove. However, these facilities, distractions and games are not always enough. It is necessary for some patients to work their way through several stages of emotional upset before they are able to utilize the recreation which is available to them.

500. Whitson, B. J. The puppet treatment in pediatrics. American Journal of Nursing, 1972, 72(9), 1612-1614.

This article describes a program at the University of South Carolina in which nursing students use hand puppets to prepare children and their families for expected surgical and nonsurgical procedures. The puppet family consists of a girl, boy, mother, father, nurse, and doctor. Construction toys, sheets, I.V. equipment, syringes, a suture set, thermometer, oxygen mask, and a doll's bed are some of the props for the puppet shows. Each show is individualized for the child to whom it is shown, so a great deal of preparation is required by the nurse acting as puppeteer. A script used for presentation to one patient is included in this article.

501. Wilkes, J. R. Don't forget the children. Canadian Medical Association Journal, 1976, 115(6), 528-529.

Serious illness or hospitalization of a parent is potentially destructive to the mental health of the child. Stress is caused by both the separation and the illness itself. If the physician does not ensure that the situation is explained to the child, it is likely the child will be confused and frightened and any attempts at clarification will be blocked in the attendant family dysfunction. The general principles of prevention are to share the facts of the situation with the child and to allow him his natural and varied reactions. The family interview is useful in clearing up misunderstandings, shared feelings and working out family roles.

502. Williams, P. D. Children's concepts of illness and internal body parts. Maternal-Child Nursing Journal, 1979, 8(2), 115-123.

This article describes a study about what hospitalized and well children know about illness and about parts inside their bodies, and what variables significantly influence knowledge of these topics. Among the findings were the following: (1) The hospitalized children knew significantly more about illness than the well children, but their knowledge of internal body parts was not significantly different; (2) On the whole, four variables significantly influenced knowledge of body parts and of illness, namely, child's grade level, father's education, mother's education, and child's sex; (3) Place of residence and mother's occupation significantly affected the scores only of well children; (4) Type of illness explained and history of illness significantly affected the scores of hospitalized children only; and (5) Ordinal position and family size significantly affected neither the well nor the hospitalized children's knowledge of illness and the body.

503. Williams, T. K. Infants' reactions to restraint of motility: A review of the literature. Maternal-Child Nursing Journal, 1973, 2 (3), 229-235.

It is generally agreed that gross muscle activity is a preferred channel for aggressive energies as well as a means of tension discharge. The first two sections of this review present some of the developmental characteristics of motility and a description of the components of the motor urge. The third section focuses on some of the reactions an infant might demonstrate when his motor urge is restricted.

504. Williams, T. K. Responses of a twelve month old girl to physical restraint during hospitalization. Maternal-Child Nursing Journal, 1975, 4(2), 109-116.

This article discusses the reactions of a 12-month-old female in terms of aggressive responses in the pre- and postoperative periods, and the reappearance of aggressive responses in the postoperative period. Observations indicate that the subject's behavior represented an aggressive fighting response to restraint. Motivated by an increase in her motor urge, she aggressively explored the various objects and people who limited her motility. When overwhelmed by restraint or debilitating illness along with restraint, she regressed to an earlier level of behavior in an effort to protect her ego against assault. Both her aggressive and regressive responses evidence unneutralized tension.

505. Willis, R. W. Happy hour: Sensitizing those who serve. Journal of the Association for the Care of Children in Hospitals, 1978, 6 (2), 17-20.

This article discusses how entertainment and activity programs offered by chaplains and by volunteers can help children cope with the common stresses and conflicts engendered by the experience of hospitalization. Examples of how these various programs can be helpful are outlined.

506. Wolfer, J. A., & Visintainer, M. A. Prehospital psychological preparation for tonsillectomy patients: Effects on children's and parents' adjustment. Pediatrics, 1979, 64(5), 646-655.

This experiment tested the stress-reducing effects of written and illustrated materials which were designed to prepare children for hospitalization for minor surgery. The preparatory materials incorporated information and procedures used successfully in previous studies to prepare children and parents in the hospital. One hundred sixty-three children three to 12 years of age and hospitalized for tonsillectomies were randomly assigned to one of five experimental groups or a control group. The experimental groups consisted of combinations of home preparation with different types of in-hospital preparation and supportive care. Children's hospital adjustment was measured by blind ratings of behavioral upset and cooperation during the blood test, medication injection, transport to surgery, induction and postoperative fluid intake. Recovery room medications and time to first voiding were also used as indications of upset. Posthospital adjustment was assessed by the Vernon _et al_. Posthospital Adjustment Inventory. Parent outcome measures included self-ratings for anxiety and satisfaction with information and care. The results indicated that children who used the home-preparatory materials alone or in combination with in-hospital preparation showed better adjustment than children in the control group. In-hospital preparation was as effective as home preparation alone or in combination with hospital preparation. Parents reported more satisfaction and less anxiety when they received some in-hospital preparation than with home preparation alone.

507. Wolfer, J. A., & Visintainer, M. A. Pediatric surgical patients' and parents' stress responses and adjustment. _Nursing Research_, 1975, _24_(4), 244-255.

The purpose of this study was to test the hypotheses that children who receive systematic psychologic preparation and continued supportive care, in contrast to those who do not, would show less upset behavior and more cooperation in the hospital and fewer posthospital adjustment problems and that their parents would be less anxious and more satisfied with information and care received. Eighty children scheduled for minor surgery and their parents were randomly assigned to experimental and control conditions. The experimental intervention consisted of accurate information about sequences of events, sensory experiences, role expectations and appropriate responses, previews of procedures through play techniques, and supportive care given at critical points pre- and postoperatively. Significant differences between experimental and control children and parents on ratings of upset behavior, cooperation with procedures, pulse before and after painful procedures, resistance to induction, time to first voiding, posthospital adjustment, and parental anxiety and satisfaction with information and care consistently supported the hypotheses. Results were also analyzed in relation to the age and sex of the children and whether parents roomed with the children.

508. Wolfgang, C. H., & Bolig, R. Play techniques for helping preschool children under stress. Journal of the Association for the Care of Children in Hospitals, 1979, 7(3), 3-10.

It is the purpose of this paper to outline a program of intervention during play based on known principles and theory of child development. The program of intervention accepts the premise that through the use of appropriate materials and teacher intervention we can recapitulate and take the nonplayers through earlier stages of play forms until they are able to accomplish higher forms of expressive play, and, in turn, re-enter the social world with others. The techniques are an expanded version of an intervention program used with autistic children (Mahler, 1970). The nonplayers, however, should not be considered pathological, nor should the techniques proposed be considered as "play therapy," but rather as facilitation of play with normal, nonplaying children who are not playing because of the situation in which they find themselves. The general purpose in a program of play intervention is to reactivate such "shut off" children and help them to acquire the ability to use their world creatively.

509. Wolinsky, G. F., & Koehler, N. A cooperative program in materials development for very young hospitalized chidlren. Rehabilitation Literature, 1973, 34(2), 34-41, 46.

This article provides a resource guide for those interested in materials and toys useful with hospitalized children functioning below their chronological age level or because of certain physical problems, need materials that are geared for a much younger group. The authors first outline how the development of materials developed and then provide a listing of suggested items.

510. Wolinsky, G. F. Materials to prepare children for hospital experiences. Exceptional Children, 1971, 37(7), 527-528.

Although the amount of time children with handicapping conditions stay in hospitals has been drastically reduced, the prospect of going to a hospital remains a rather frightening experience for both the child and the family. This article presents a selection of printed materials that have been developed by various hospitals and nonprofit organizations to help in explaining to the child what a hospital stay actually means. While acquainting the child through this rather elementary way with the meaning of his projected hospital stay does not immediately ensure that the child will still not be anxious or fearful, it does offer a child an opportunity to explore his own anxieties and fantasies. The materials were chosen because they are inexpensive and can be given to individual children for personal use. They can also be of value to teachers working with children who face a series of operations during their early years of life.

511. Woods, L. G. Dominant coping behaviors of a hospitalized four year old deaf boy. Maternal-Child Nursing Journal, 1979, 8(3), 181-193.

This article presents the case study of a deaf four year old boy, Matthew, hospitalized for a repeat release of the Achilles tendon. During his hospital stay, three mechanisms were used predominantly by Matthew to cope with his experience. They were (1) information gathering, (2) avoidance, and (3) comfort seeking behaviors. Matthew's behavior during his hospitalization demonstrated the way in which he reorganized his senses to compensate for his hearing loss and to cope with the stress caused by hospital experiences. His vision was used constantly as a background lead sense; it was used as the foreground sense when his scanning detected a potential source of threat. His sense of touch was utilized as a foreground sense as Matthew gradually became more comfortable with his surroundings. It also served as a source of comfort from his mother. Avoidance of stimuli to delay intake of unpleasant information was practiced with both vision and touch. By compensating for his auditory deprivation with greater reliance on remaining senses, Matthew coped with the hospitalization in a successful manner.

512. Young, M. Children in hospital: Caring for the needs of the child and the family. Nursing Times, 1979, 75(18), 740-741.

This article describes care in the children's wards at The Royal National Orthopedic Hospital in England. Careful preparation of children before admission, and individualized care during their stay can help them cope with separation from their families. By taking time to think about the children's and parents' feelings, as well as arranging group discussions, the staff have deepened their awareness of the pain of separation, the stress of a hospital stay, and the dangers to the child of maternal deprivation. They have become more alert to recognizing the signs of behavior disturbance. Their philosophy is illustrated by describing the care of a child from the outpatient department until discharged, and suggestions for ways in which to prepare the child for hospitalization are presented.

513. Zide, B., & Pardoe, R. The use of behavior modification therapy in a recalcitrant burned child. Plastic and Reconstructive Surgery, 1976, 57(3), 378-382.

The hospital behavior of a burned adolescent is presented, with emphasis on the antecedent causes. The authors used a behavior modification technique to treat this patient, and this article describes the basic characteristics of this procedure. Environmental procedures were used to control the consequences of the patient's voluntary behavior. Ultimately, the patient was able to control the consequences himself. The target set of behaviors to be modified (i.e., eating, physical therapy, dressing changes, and general attitude) was identified. A set of rewards was then devised to "control" this behavior. He became constructive rather than self-destructive, and he learned to cope with the discomforts because of the satisfying outcomes. The situation was manipulated to influence his behavior; in this way, his in-hospital life was made happier and more enjoyable.

514. Zweig, I. K. A new way to get acquainted with the hospital--Pediatric open house for well children. MCN: American Journal of Maternal Child Nursing, 1976, 1(4), 217-219.

This article discusses a new way to help parents and children cope with a hospital experience. Rahway Hospital instituted a Pediatric Open House program for the well child and his parents to acquaint the community with Rahway Hospital, the people who work there, and some hospital procedures. At the present time the program is held two Sundays a month. The children, either accompanied by their parents or attending with a local organization, assemble in a conference room. Two nurses, a unit clerk, and candy stripers from the pediatric and adolescent unit greet the members of the group, all of whom have been given a hospital name bracelet. The community's response to it has been excellent. Many letters have been received thanking the hospital and its staff for making hospitalization a less frightening experience for the child and his parents.

LATE ADDITIONS

The following references were obtained too late to be verified and abstracted. They are listed here as an additional source of information regarding childhood experiences with hospitalization.

1. Anderson, E. G. The child in hospital: Play and emotional needs. Australasian Nurses Journal, 1978, 7, 54-57.

2. Anonymous. Children's hospital philosophy. Australasian Nurses Journal, 1975, 3(10), 8, 29.

3. Barker, P. Psychological effects on children of admission to hospital. Update, 1974, 9(8), 1019-1024.

4. Brennan, A. Preoperative play cart. Orthopedic Nurses Association Journal, 1978, 5(1), 21-22.

5. Brian, J. Child's play. Midwife, Health Visitor and Community Nurse, 1977, 13(6), 182-185.

6. Burch, G. E. The cruelities in the practice of medicine. American Health Journal, 1974, 87, 800.

7. Caroll, E. The welfare of children in hospital. Australasian Nurses Journal, 1977, 7, 39-41.

8. Chan, J. M. Preparation for hospitalization, procedures and surgery through play. Australasian Nurses Journal, 1976, 5(4), 41-44.

9. Cook, A. Play schemes for children in hospitals. Midwife, Health Visitor and Community Nurse, 1978, 14(3), 82-83.

10. Crocker, E. Is your hospital any place for a three-year-old? Dimensions of Health Service, 1975, 52(7), 32-33.

11. Dicken, K. Unrestricted visiting in children's wards--how is it working out? Midwife Health Visit, 1971, 7, 185-187.

12. Endres, G. Maternal deprivation and role playing of the hospitalized child. Journal of New York State Nurses Association, 1974, 5, 17-19.

13. Fowler, J. The emotional care of the burned child. Australasian Nurses Journal, 1977, 7(3), 13-15.

14. Green, J. R. Planning for play in hospital. Australasian Nurses Journal, 1976, 5(4), 10-12.

15. Gruber, D. L. Helping the child accept I.V. therapy. American Journal of IV Therapy, 1977, 4, 50-51.

16. Hardgrove, C. Care through parent program. Australasian Nurses Journal, 1975, 3(10), 8.

17. Hart, D. Role of play leader in hospital. Australasian Nurses Journal, 1976, 5(4), 30-32.

18. Harvey, S. Play for children in hospitals. International Journal of Early Childhood, 1975, 7(2), 185-187.

19. Hunter, P. A program of integrated hospital and home nursing care for children. Australasian Nurses Journal, 1975, 3(10), 12-13.

20. Iodice, C. From the child's point of view. Health Care Education, 1977, 6, 24-26.

21. James, J. Play for children in hospital. Australasian Nurses Journal, 1976, 5(4), 33-35.

22. Kearns, T. The psychology of play. Australasian Nurses Journal, 1976, 5(4), 25-26.

23. Koperno, M. Play is not enough. Australasian Nurses Journal, 1976, 5(4), 57-58.

24. Koperno, M. Meeting the emotional needs of young children and their families. Australasian Nurses Journal, 1977, 6(11), 17-20.

25. Langley, E. M. Play and the hospitalized child. Australasian Nurses Journal, 1976, 5(4), 40-41.

26. Miles, M. S. Impact of the intensive care unit on parents. Issues in Comprehensive Pediatric Nursing, 1979, 3(7), 72-90.

27. Morris, D. The pediatrician and play in the hospital. Australasian Nurses Journal, 1976, 5(4), 49-50.

28. Parsonage, S. Preparation of children going into hospitals. District Nurse, 1971, 14, 30.

29. Pinkus, S. Going into hospital. New York: International Publications Service, 1973.

30. Prugh, D. G., & Jordan, K. Physical illness or injury: The hospital as a source of emotional disturbances in child and family. In I. Berlin (Ed.), Advocacy for child mental health. New York: Brunner/Mazel, 1975, 208-249.

31. Raikes, A. S. Importance of play in hospital. Australasian Nurses Journal, 1976, 5(4), 45-48.

32. Rankin, C. Toys and activities for play in hospital. Australasian Nurses Journal, 1976, 5(4), 17-23.

33. Rustin, T. A. Caring for the emotional needs of hospitalized children: How sophomore students can help. The New Physician, 1972, March, 136-139.

34. Sainsbury, E. Music and play in hospital. Australasian Nurses Journal, 1976, 5(4), 28-29.

35. Sarles, R. M. The use of hypnosis with hospitalized children. Journal of Clinical Child Psychiatry, 1975, 4, 36-38.

36. Smith, L. G. Preparing a child for hospital stay--a community project. Canadian Hospital, 1971, 48, 46-48.

37. Southard, S. C. Summary report of the expert group on play for children in hospitals department of health and social security. Journal of Advanced Nursing, 1976, 1(5), 425-428.

38. Weller, J. E. Bibliotherapy for children. Canadian Journal of Psychiatric Nursing, 1977, 18(4), 9-13.

39. Wieczorek, R. Children's art: The comparison of drawings of hospitalized and non-hospitalized five to seven year olds. Journal of New York State Nurses Association, 1974, 5, 20-26.

40. Williams, J. R. Parent participation. Australasian Nurses Journal, 1975, 3(10), 26.

41. Wood, N. Conditioning parents and children for hospital. Australasian Nurses Journal, 1976, 5(4), 36, 62.

HISTORICAL REFERENCES (1960-1969)

The following references published in the 1960's represent additional information about the ill and hospitalized child. Because of the great number of these references, they are presented here in citation form only, without abstracts.

1. Abruzzi, W. Are hospitals ruining your children? Medical Times, 1966, 94(12), 1439-1443.

2. Adams, M. L., & Berman, D. C. The hospital through a child's eyes. Children, 1965, 12, 102-104.

3. Aldrich, R. A. Pediatrics--Its present and future. In M. F. Shore (Ed.), Red is the color of hurting. Washington, D. C.: Government Printing Office, 1965, 5-14.

4. Ambler, M. C. Disciplining hospitalized toddlers. American Journal of Nursing, 1967, 67, 572-573.

5. Amend, E. L. Orientation for the short-term surgical patient. In B. S. Bergersen, E. H. Anderson, M. Duffey, M. Lohr and M. H. Rose (Eds.), Current concepts in clinical nursing, Volume II. St. Louis: C. V. Mosby Company, 1969, 230-236.

6. Ammon, K. J. The effects of music on children in respiratory distress. ANA clinical sessions, 1968, Dallas. New York: Appleton-Century-Crofts, 1968, 127-133.

7. Anonymous. Care of children in hospitals. Evanston, Illinois: American Academy of Pediatrics, 1960.

8. Anonymous. Viewpoints on children in hospitals: The children. Hospitals, 1963, 37, 43-46.

9. Anonymous. Credo on the needs of the hospitalized child. Nursing Outlook, 1966, 14, 41.

10. Anonymous. Cause for concern. British Medical Journal, 1969, 4 701.

11. Anonymous. A child in hospital. Lancet, 1969, 1, 413.

12. Anonymous. Children in hospital: Ten years of progress. British Hospital Journal, 1969, 79, 2378.

13. Anonymous. Mothers in hospital. Lancet, 1969, 2, 580.

14. Arenson, S. A. Changes in a toddler's mode of adapting to separation from his mother during daily relationship experiences with one nurse. ANA clinical sessions, 1968, Dallas. New York: Appleton-Century-Crofts, 1968, 134-141.

15. Aufhauser, T. R. Parent participation in hospital care of children. Nursing Outlook, 1967, 15(1), 40-42.

16. Bailey, T. F. Puppets teach young patients. Nursing Outlook, 1967, 15, 36-37.

17. Barton, P. H. Play as a tool of nursing. Nursing Outlook, 1962, 10(3), 162-164.

18. Barton, P. H. The relationship between fantasy and overt stress reactions of children to hospitalization (Doctoral dissertation, University of Florida, 1964). Dissertation Abstracts International, 1968, 29(3-A), 809.

19. Barton, P. H. Nursing assessment and intervention through play. In B. S. Bergerson, E. H. Anderson, M. Duffey, M. Lohr and M. H. Rose (Eds.), Current concepts in clinical nursing, Volume II. St. Louis: C. V. Mosby Company, 1969, 203-217.

20. Bavin, J. T. Children in adult wards. British Medical Journal, 1968, 4, 576-577.

21. Belmont, H. S. The child patient. GP, 1963, 28, 82-89.

22. Bergmann, T. Children in the hospital. New York: International Universities Press, Inc., 1965.

23. Bernstein, N. R., Sanger, S., & Fras, I. The functions of the child psychiatrist in the management of severely burned children. Journal of the American Academy of Child Psychiatry, 1969, 8(4), 620-636.

24. Best, B. M. Children's reactions to hospital: A survey. Nursing Times, 1963, 59, 1492-1493.

25. Beurke, P. Educational programming for the short term hospitalized child. Exceptional Children, 1966, 32, 559-563.

26. Bielicka, I., & Olechnowicz, H. Treating children traumatized by hospitalization. Children, 1963, 10(5), 194-195.

27. Blake, F. G. Immobilized youth: A rationale for supportive nursing intervention. American Journal of Nursing, 1969, 69(11), 2364-2369.

28. Blatherwick, C. E. The paediatric orientation-to-hospital program. Alberta Medical Bulletin, 1969, 34(1), 12-16.

29. Bliss, B. Going to the hospital--a child's eye view. Hospital Topics, 1967, 45, 30-31.

30. Blumgart, E., & Korsch, B. M. Pediatric recreation: An approach to meeting the emotional needs of hospitalized children. Pediatrics, 1964, 34(1), 133-136.

31. Bodeker, M. P. Nursing services in a children's hospital. In M. F. Shore (Ed.), Red is the color of hurting. Washington, D. C.: United States Government Printing Office, 1965, 37-44.

32. Bongiovanni, A. M. Hospitalization of children: Report of an international seminar. Pediatrics, 1964, 34(1), 1-3.

33. Bonnem, S. Out-of-univorm nurses make hit with kids. Modern Hospital, 1967, 108, 90.

34. Borenz, H. F. Children's personality reaction to chronic illness. The Wisconsin Medical Journal, 1962, 61(11), 551-554.

35. Bowley, A. H. The psychological care of the child in hospital. Edinburgh: E. & S. Livingstone, Ltd., 1961.

36. Brain, D. J., & Maclay, I. Controlled study of mothers and children in hospital. British Medical Journal, 1968, 1(5587), 278-280.

37. Branstetter, E. The young child's response to hospitalization: Separation anxiety or lack of mothering care? American Journal of Public Health, 1969, 59(1), 92-97.

38. Branstetter, E. The young child's response to hospitalization: Separation anxiety or lack of mothering care? Communicating Nursing Research, 1969, 2, 13-25.

39. Branstetter, E. Response to critique: "The young child's response to hospitalization: Separation anxiety or lack of mothering care?" Communicating Nursing Research, 1969, 2, 41-44.

40. Briggs, R. F. The emotional needs of children in hospital. Canadian Medical Association Journal, 1966, 94(10), 485-487.

41. Briggs, R. F. The hospitalized child faces emotional hazards. Hospital Management, 1967, 103(5), 90-92.

42. Brodie, B., & Matern, S. Emotional aspects in the care of a severely burned girl. International Nursing Review, 1967, 14(6), 19-24.

43. Brooks, M. Play for hospitalized children. Young Children, 1969, 24, 224.

44. Brotherton, M. G. Nurse-parent-patient relations. In B. S. Bergersen, E. H. Anderson, M. Duffey, M. Lohr and M. H. Rose (Eds.), Current concepts in clinical nursing, Volume II. St. Louis: C. V. Mosby Company, 1969, 237-239.

45. Buckley, H. E. A description and criticism of an audio-visual presentation for children facing hospitalization (Doctoral dissertation, Columbia University, 1962). Dissertation Abstracts International, 1963, 23(11), 4254-4255.

46. Burling, K. A., & Collipp, P. J. Emotional responses of hospitalized children: Results of a pulse-monitor study. Clinical Pediatrics, 1969, 8, 641-646.

47. Byers, M. L. The hospitalized adolescent. Nursing Outlook, 1967, 15(8), 32-34.

48. Cassell, S. E. The effects of brief puppet therapy upon the emotional responses of children undergoing cardiac catheterization (Doctoral dissertation, Northwestern University, 1963). Dissertation Abstracts International, 1964, 25(3), 2042.

49. Cassell, S., & Paul, M. H. The role of puppet therapy on the emotional responses of children hospitalized for cardiac catheterization. Journal of Pediatrics, 1967, 71(2), 233-239.

50. Chambers, P., Dutson, C., Burke, A., & Gunby, G. The adolescent in hospital. Nursing Times, 1968, 64(37), 1240-1241.

51. Cohen, R., Alle, R., & Band, P. Reaching the hospitalized child through recreational therapy. Nursing Clinics of North America, 1966, 1, 73.

52. Coleman, L. L. Psychological preparation of the child for surgery. In H. I. Lief, V. F. Lief, and N. R. Lief (Eds.), The psychological basis of medical practice. New York: Harper & Row Publishers, Inc., 1963, 362-369.

53. Condon, M., & Peters, C. Family participation unit. American Journal of Nursing, 1968, 68(3), 504-507.

54. Cooke, R. E. Effects of hospitalization upon the child. In J. A. Haller, Jr. (Ed.), The hospitalized child and his family. Baltimore: Johns Hopkins Press, 1967, 3-17.

55. Coughlan, C. J. The child for surgery. The prevention of psychological upsets. East African Medical Journal, 1965, 42, 32-41.

56. Daubenmire, M. J., Pierce, L. M., & Weaver, B. R. Adolescence in the hospital. Nursing Outlook, 1960, 8(9), 502-504.

57. David, M., & Appell, G. A study of nursing care and nurse-infant interaction. In B. M. Foss (Ed.), Determinants of infant behaviour, Volume I. New York: John Wiley & Sons, Inc., 1961, 121-141.

58. Davis, E. L. Play interviews used to evaluate a child's reaction to hospitalization. Hospital Topics, 1961, September, 61.

59. Denyes, M. J. A child with Hirschsprung's disease uses a nurse to gain ego strength. ANA clinical sessions, 1968, Dallas. New York: Appleton-Century-Crofts, 1968, 155-161.

60. Dimock, H. G. The child in hospital: A study of his emotional and social well-being. Philadelphia: F. A. Davis Company, 1960.

61. Dittmann, L. L. A child's sense of trust. American Journal of Nursing, 1966, 66, 91-93.

62. Dombro, R. H. Child Life Programs in ninety-one children's hospitals in the United States and Canada. In J. A. Haller, Jr. (Ed.), The hospitalized child and his family. Baltimore: John Hopkins Press, 1967, 89-102.

63. Dombro, R. H. Child Life Programs in ninety-two pediatric departments of general hospitals in the United States and Canada. In J. A. Haller, Jr. (Ed.), The hospitalized child and his family. Baltimore: Johns Hopkins Press, 1967, 105-117.

64. Dombro, R. H., & Haas, B. S. The Helen Schnetzer Child Life Program. In J. A. Haller, Jr. (Ed.), The hospitalized child and his family. Baltimore: John Hopkins Press, 1967, 79-86.

65. Duncombe, M. A. Visiting children in hospital. International Nursing Review, 1966, 13(3), 32-36.

66. Englebardt, S. L. Care-by-parent relieves emotional strain on children, financial strain on parents. Modern Hospital, 1969, 113 (6), 94-97.

67. Erickson, F. View points on children in hospitals: Nurse. Hospitals, 1963, 37, 47-48.

68. Erickson, F. When 6- to 12- year olds are ill. Nursing Outlook, 1965, 13, 48-50.

69. Erickson, F. H. Helping the sick child maintain behavioral control. Nursing Clinics of North America, 1967, 2(4), 695-703.

70. Erickson, F. Nursing care based on nursing assessment. In B. S. Bergersen, E. H. Anderson, M. Duffey, M. Lohr and M. H. Rose (Eds.), Current concepts in clinical nursing, Volume II. St. Louis: C. V. Mosby Company, 1969, 171-177.

71. Esslinger, P. N. Challenge and problems of helping auxiliary personnel understand and work with children. In B. S. Bergersen, E. H. Anderson, M. Duffey, M. Lohr and M. H. Rose (Eds.), Current concepts in clinical nursing, Volume II. St. Louis: C. V. Mosby Company, 1969, 240-248.

72. Fagin, C. M. Why not involve parents when children are hospitalized? American Journal of Nursing, 1962, 62(6), 78-79.

73. Fagin, C. M. The case for rooming in when young children are hospitalized. Nursing Science, 1964, 2, 323-333.

74. Fagin, C. M. Rooming in and its effects on the behavior of young children: A comparative survey on the effects of maternal attendance during hospitalization on the post hospital behavior of young children (Doctoral dissertation, New York University, 1964). Dissertation Abstracts International, 1965, 25(8), 4657-4658.

75. Fagin, C. M. Effects of maternal attendance during hospitalization on the post-hospital behaviour of young children. Philadelphia: F. A. Davis, 1966.

76. Fagin, C. M. Pediatric rooming-in: Its meaning for the nurse. Nursing Clinics of North America, 1966, 1(1), 83-93.

77. Fagin, C. M. Therapeutic intervention with adolescents--the nurse and the adolescent. In B. S. Bergersen, E. H. Anderson, M. Duffey, M. Lohr and M. H. Rose (Eds.), Current concepts in clinical nursing, Volume II. St. Louis: C. V. Mosby Company, 1969, 116-125.

78. Faigel, H. C. The hospitalized child. Connecticut Medicine, 1966, 30(11), 796-798.

79. Fineberg, H. H., & Jone, E. C. Mother bank in a children's hospital. Journal of the American Medical Association, 1960, 174(17), 2153-2154.

80. Flandorf, V. S. Preparing a child for hospitalization. GP, 1965, 31(3), 107-110.

81. Freilich, H. Psychologic problems in hospitalization of children. Hospital Topics, 1966, 44(2), 103-105.

82. Galdston, R., & Gamble, W. J. On borrowed time: Observations on children with implanted cardiac pacemakers and their families. American Journal of Psychiatry, 1969, 126(1), 104-108.

83. Geis, D. P. Home visits help prepare preschoolers and their parents for hospitalization. ANA regional clinical conferences, 1967, Philadelphia/Kansas City. New York: Appleton-Century-Crofts, 1968, 180-188.

84. Geis, D. P., & Rochon, D. Home visits help prepare preschoolers for hospital experience. Hospitals, 1966, 40(4), 83, 86-87.

85. Geist, H. A child goes to the hospital: The psychological aspects of a child going to the hospital. Springfield, Illinois: Charles C. Thomas, 1965.

86. Goldman, H. B., & Bohcali, A. Psychologic preparation of children for tonsillectomy. Laryngoscope, 1966, 76(10), 1698-1705.

87. Green, M. A new arrangement for hospital services: The parent-care pavilion. Pediatrics, 1969, 43(4, part 1), 486-487.

88. Green, M., & Segar, W. E. A new design for patient care and pediatric education in a children's hospital: An interim report. Pediatrics, 1961, 28(5), 825-837.

89. Hadley, B. J. Becoming well: A study of role change (Doctoral disseration, University of California, Los Angeles, 1966). Dissertation Abstracts International, 1966, 26(11), 6905-6906.

90. Haggerty, A. M. Approaches to coping with adolescents. ANA clinical sessions, 1966, San Francisco. New York: Appleton-Century-Crofts, 1967, 151-156.

91. Hales-Tooke, A. Improving hospital care for children. Children, 1968, 15(3), 116-118.

92. Haller, J. A., Jr. Preparing a child for his operation. In J. A. Haller, Jr. (Ed.), The hospitalized child and his family. Baltimore: Johns Hopkins Press, 1967, 19-31.

93. Hammon, J. The preparation of the pediatric patient for hospital school--a pilot study. Journal of School Health, 1967, 37, 459-464.

94. Healy, K. M. Does preoperative instruction make a difference? American Journal of Nursing, 1968, 68, 62-67.

95. Heavenrich, R. M. Viewpoints on children in hospitals. Hospitals, 1963, 37, 40-42.

96. Hillman, S. Adolescents' reactions to hospitalization. Henry Ford Hospital Medical Bulletin, 1962, 10, 443-444.

97. Holt, J. L. Children's recall of a pre-school age hospital experience after an interval of five years (Doctoral dissertation, University of Pittsburgh, 1967). Dissertation Abstracts International, 1968, 28(8-B), 3352.

98. Holt, J. L. Discussion of the method and the clinical implications from the study "Children's recall of a pre-school age hospital experience after an interval of five years." In M. V. Batey (Ed.), Communicating nursing research. Boulder, Colorado: Western Interstate Commission for Higher Education, 1968, 56-72.

99. Hopkins, J. Children in hospital: Observations on the reactions of Chinese children to hospitalization with implications for child care practices. Far East Medical Journal, 1969, 5, 279-284.

100. Howe, J. Children's ideas about injury. ANA regional clinical conferences, 1967, Philadelphia/Kansas City. New York: Appleton-Century-Crofts, 1968, 189-195.

101. Hughes, R. B. Children's fears of surgery. Hospital Topics, 1967, 45(9), 116-117.

102. Jacoby, N. M. Unrestricted visiting in a children's ward: The first twenty years. Lancet, 1969, 2, 584-586.

103. James, F. E. The behaviour reactions of normal children to common operations. Practitioner, 1960, 185(1106), 339-342.

104. Johnson, M. E. Preparation of infants, children for cardiac catheterization. Hospital Topics, 1968, 46, 67-69.

105. Jolly, H. Play and the sick child: A comparative study of its role in a teaching hospital in London and one in Ghana. Lancet, 1968, 2, 1286-1287.

106. Jolly, H. Play is work: The role of play for sick and healthy children. Lancet, 1969, 2, 487-488.

107. Kangery, R. H. Children's answers. American Journal of Nursing, 1960, 60(12), 1748-1751.

108. Katcher, A. L., & Grant, E. V. Parents help care for their children. Hospitals, 1961, 35(5), 83-86.

109. Kazan, A. T., Browning, T. B., & Cohen, A. D. Emotional implications of child care practices on pediatric units of general hospitals in Westchester County: Survey and recommendations. New York State Journal of Medicine, 1965, 65, 2568-2572.

110. Katz, G. Mothers help care for sick children in experimental unit. Hospitals, 1964, 38(13), 38-42.

111. Kennedy, D. A. Planning a new children's hospital. In M. F. Shore (Ed.), Red is the color of hurting. Washington, D. C.: United States Government Printing Office, 1965, 63-70.

112. Korsch, B. M. Psychological reactions to physical illness in children. Journal of the Medical Association of Georgia, 1961, 50 (11), 519-523.

113. Kravitz, H. Hospitalization of children as a psychological benefit and learning experience. Illinois Medical Journal, 1965, 127, 380.

114. Kravitz, H. Survey of visiting privileges for pediatric patients in hospitals. Illinois Medical Journal, 1969, 135, 597-599.

115. Kresky, B., & Simon, B. E. Infantile reaction to facial disfigurement. Archives of Surgery, 1961, 82, 783-788.

116. Kuenssberg, C. V. When Bruce goes to hospital (at the age of four years). Nursing Times, 1964, 60, 688-690.

117. Langford, W. S. The child in the pediatric hospital: Adaptation to illness and hospitalization. American Journal of Orthopsychiatry, 1961, 31, 667-684.

118. Lawrie, R. Operating on children as day-cases. Lancet, 1964, 2, 1289-1291.

119. Laybourne, P. C., & Miller, H. C. Pediatric hospitalization of psychiatric patients: Diagnostic and therapeutic implications. American Journal of Orthopsychiatry, 1962, 32(4), 596-603.

120. Lee, J. S., & Greene, N. M. Parental presence and emotional state of children prior to surgery. Clinical Pediatrics, 1969, 8(3), 126-130.

121. Leininger, M. Critique: The young child's response to hospitalization: Separation anxiety or lack of mothering care? Communicating Nursing Research, 1969, 2, 26-40.

122. Leman, E. Mothers make effective aides at Hunterdon Medical Center. Hospital Topics, 1966, 44, 95-98.

123. Lemkau, P. The importance of play for the child in the hospital. In J. A. Haller, Jr. (Ed.), The hospitalized child and his family. Baltimore: Johns Hopkins Press, 1967, 43-51.

124. LeRoux, R., & Arlton, D. The foster grandparent program. Nursing Forum, 1969, 8(4), 405-415.

125. Lipton, H. Pre-school activities program within a medical framework. Canadian Hospital, 1968, 45, 54-58.

126. Lipton, S. D. On the psychology of childhood tonsillectomy. Psychoanalytic Study of the Child, 1962, 17, 363-417.

127. Little, S. Psychology of physical illness in adolescents. Pediatric Clinics of North America, 1960, 7(1), 85-96.

128. Long, R. T., & Cope, O. Emotional problems of burned children. New England Journal of Medicine, 1961, 264(22), 1121-1127.

129. Loomis, W. G. The use of a foster grandmother in the psychotherapy of a preschool child on a pediatric ward. Clinical Pediatrics, 1967, 6(7), 384-386.

130. Lynn, H. B. Details that count in the surgical care of children. American Journal of Surgery, 1961, 101, 553-561.

131. MacCarthy, D., Lindsay, M., & Morris, I. Children in hospital with mothers. Lancet, 1962, 1, 603-608.

132. MacDonald, E. M. Parents participate in care of the hospitalized child. Canadian Nurse, 1969, 65, 37-39.

133. MacKeith, A. The involvement of the hospital staff with the child in hospital, or empathy in the hospital. Bibliotheca Paediatrica, 1965, 84, 183-189.

134. Mahaffy, P. R., Jr. The effects of hospitalization on children admitted for tonsillectomy and adenoidectomy. Nursing Research, 1965, 14(1), 12-19.

135. Martin, R. L. The acute situational crisis and communication theory (Doctoral dissertation, University of Southern California, 1968). Dissertation Abstracts International, 1968, 29(4-A), 1296.

136. Mason, E. A. The hospitalized child: His emotional needs. New England Journal of Medicine, 1965, 272, 406-414.

137. Mayer, J. Reactions of children during hospital admission: Three diaries. Mental Hygiene, 1964, 48, 576-580.

138. McCaffery, M. Brief episodes of pain in children. In B. S. Bergersen, E. H. Anderson, M. Duffey, M. Lohr and M. H. Rose (Eds.), Current concepts in clinical nursing, Volume II. St. Louis: C. V. Mosby Company, 1969, 178-191.

139. McClure, M. J. Care-by-parent unit. American Journal of Nursing, 1969, 69, 2248-2152.

140. McCranie, M. S. Reducing emotional trauma from elective surgery of children. Journal of the Medical Association of Georgia, 1962, 51, 222-225.

141. McGhee, S. D. The mother-complement role of the nurse in family centered child care. Hospital Progress, 1968, 49, 94, 96.

142. McGurn, W. C. Supportive nursing care as a means of promoting the independence of an adolescent boy having open heart surgery. ANA clinical sessions, 1966, San Francisco. New York: Appleton-Century-Crofts, 1967, 46-53.

143. McPherson, C. A. The value of play in meeting the emotional needs of young children in hospital. Bibliotheca Paediatrica, 1965, 84, 181-182.

144. Meadow, S. R. Mothers and children in hospital. British Medical Journal, 1968, 2, 560.

145. Meadow, S. R. The captive mother. Archives of Disease in Childhood, 1969, 44, 362-367.

146. Meagher, M. Family-centered pediatrics. Hospital Progress, 1967, 48, 100-102.

147. Mechanic, D. The influence of mothers on their children's health attitudes and behavior. Pediatrics, 1964, 33(3), 444-453.

148. Mellish, R. W. P. Preparation of a child for hospitalization and surgery. Pediatric Clinics of North America, 1969, 16(3), 543-553.

149. Merrow, D. L., & Johnson, B. Perceptions of the mother's role with her hospitalized child. Nursing Research, 1968, 17(2), 155-156.

150. Meyer, H. L. Predictable problems of hospitalized adolescents. American Journal of Nursing, 1969, 69(3), 525-528.

151. Micic, Z. Psychological stress in children in hospital. International Nursing Review, 1962, 9(6), 23-31.

152. Minde, K., & Maler, L. Psychiatric counseling on a pediatric medical ward: A controlled evaluation. Journal of Pediatrics, 1968, 72(4), 452-460.

153. Mitchell, J. V. Recreational therapy program alleviates homesickness. Hospital Topics, 1967, 45, 97-98.

154. Moncrieff, A. Human relations in child health: Children in the hospital. Journal of the Royal Institute of Public Health and Hygiene, 1963, 26(3), 57-64.

155. Moore, C., & Rose, M. H. Working with children and their families to help them through a long-anticipated surgical experience. In B. S. Bergersen, E. H. Anderson, M. Duffey, M. Lohr and M. H. Rose (Eds.), Current concepts in clinical nursing. St. Louis: C. V. Mosby Company, 1967, 311-327.

156. Moore, R. F., Albert, R. S., Manning, M. J., & Glasser, B. A. Explorations in alternatives to hospitalization. American Journal of Psychiatry, 1962, 119, 560-569.

157. Moran, P. A. Parents in pediatrics. Nursing Forum, 1963, 2(3), 24-37.

158. Morgan, B. D. Mothers in hospital. The nurses' viewpoint. Lancet, 1967, 2, 38-39.

159. Morgan, B. D. Visiting in children's units: A changing pattern. Nursing Times, 1967, 63(12), 1711-1713.

160. Morgenstern, F. S. Facilities for children's play in hospitals. Developmental Medicine and Child Neurology, 1968, 10(1), 111-114.

161. Murrin, M. A. Billy needs to play. RN, 1969, 32(12), 38-43.

162. Nealon, J. The adolescent's hospitalization as a family crisis. Implications for a therapeutic approach. Archives of General Psychology, 1964, 11, 302-311.

163. Neill, C. A. The child and his family at home after hospitalization. In J. A. Haller, Jr. (Ed.), The hospitalized child and his family. Baltimore: Johns Hopkins Press, 1967, 67-77.

164. Noble, E. The value of play for young children in hospital I. Nursing Times, 1964, 60(49), 607-608.

165. O'Connell, E. A., & Brandt, P. Liberal visiting hours for parents. American Journal of Nursing, 1960, 60, 812-815.

166. O'Grady, R. S. Restraint and the hospitalized child. In B. S. Bergersen, E. H. Anderson, M. Duffey, M. Lohr and M. H. Rose (Eds.), Current concepts in clinical nursing, Volume II. St. Louis: C. V. Mosby Company, 1969, 192-202.

167. Outland, C. A. W. A child is hospitalized. American Journal of Nursing, 1964, 64(6), 135-136.

168. Patterson, B. B., & Tarule, J. M. Working-play of the hospital child. Journal of Practical Nursing, 1966, 16(11), 25-29, 45.

169. Pavenstedt, E. A child guidance service in a municipal hospital. Children, 1963, 10(6), 207-212.

170. Pead, J. Mothers and children in hospital. British Medical Journal, 1968, 2, 303.

171. Pead, J. Overvisiting of hospital patients? Lancet, 1968, 1, 200.

172. Peay, R. The emotional problems of children facing heart surgery. Children, 1960, 7, 223-228.

173. Petrillo, M. Preventing hospital trauma in pediatric patients. American Journal of Nursing, 1968, 68(7), 1469-1473.

174. Pickett, L. K. The hospital environment for the pediatric surgical patient. Pediatric Clinics of North America, 1969, 16(3), 531-542.

175. Pidgeon, V. A. Children's concepts of the rationale of isolation technic. ANA clinical sessions, 1966, San Francisco. New York: Appleton-Century-Crofts, 1967, 21-27.

176. Pill, R. Space and social structure in two children's wards. Sociological Review, 1967, 15, 179-192.

177. Plank, E. N. Working with children in hospitals: A guide for the professional team. Cleveland: The Press of Case Western Reserve University, 1962.

178. Plank, E. N. Preparing children for surgery. The Ohio State Medical Journal, 1963, 59(8), 809-811.

179. Plank, E. N. Abandonment: Deepest fear of hospitalized children. Hospital Topics, 1965, 43(9), 93-96.

180. Post, S. Hospitalization of children under five. Canadian Nurse, 1966, 62(7), 34-37.

181. Potts, W. J. The hospitalized child. Illinois Medical Journal, 1963, 123(3), 235-239.

182. Prugh, D. G. Emotional aspects of the hospitalization of children. In M. F. Shore (Ed.), Red is the color of hurting. Washington, D. C.: United States Government Printing Office, 1965, 17-34.

183. Prugh, D. G. Children's reactions to illness, hospitalization, and surgery. In A. M. Friedman and H. I. Kaplan (Eds.), Comprehensive textbook of psychiatry. Baltimore: Williams & Wilkins Company, 1967, 1369-1375.

184. Rendle-Short, J. The child in hospital. Medical Journal of Australia, 1962, 49(17), 632-633.

185. Rie, H. E., Boverman, H., Grossman, B. J., & Ozoa, N. Immediate and long-term effects of interventions early in prolonged hospitalization. Pediatrics, 1968, 41(4), 755-764.

186. Rie, H. E., Voerman, H., Ozoa, N., & Grossman, B. J. Tutoring and ventilation: A pilot study of reactions of hospitalized children. Clinical Pediatrics, 1964, 3, 581.

187. Rieger, N. I. A community nursery school program for hospitalized children. Mental Hygiene, 1969, 53, 196-199.

188. Riley, I. D., Syme, J., Hall, M. S., & Patrick, M. J. Mother and child in hospital--two years' experience. British Medical Journal, 1965, 2(5468), 990-992.

189. Roberta, M. A doll goes to surgery. American Journal of Nursing, 1963, 63, 82.

190. Robertson, J. Hospitals and children: A parent's-eye view. New York: International Universities Press, Inc., 1962.

191. Robertson, J. Effecting change in the hospitalization of children. In M. F. Shore (Ed.), Red is the color of hurting. Washington, D. C.: United States Government Printing Office, 1965, 47-60.

192. Robinson, D. Mothers' fear, their children's well-being in hospital, and the study of illness behaviour. British Journal of Preventive and Social Medicine, 1968, 22(4), 228-233.

193. Robinson, G. C., Shah, C. P., Argue, C., Kinnis, C., & Israels, S. A study of the need for alternative types of health care for children in hospitals. Pediatrics, 1969, 43(5), 866-878.

194. Rothenberg, M. B. Child psychiatry-pediatrics liaison: A history and commentary. Journal of the American Academy of Child Psychiatry, 1968, 17(3), 492-509.

195. Rothman, P. E. A note on hospitalism. Pediatrics, 1962, 30(6), 995-999.

196. Rousseau, O. Mothers do help in pediatrics. American Journal of Nursing, 1967, 67(4), 798-800.

197. Roy, M. C. Role cues and mothers of hospitalized children. Nursing Research, 1967, 16(2), 178-182.

198. Roy, M. C. Role cues for the mother of the hospitalized child. ANA clinical sessions, 1968, Dallas. New York: Appleton-Century-Crofts, 1968, 199-206.

199. Rubin, M. Caring for children with illnesses requiring long-term hospitalization. In B. S. Bergersen, E. H. Anderson, M. Duffey, M. Lohr and M. H. Rose (Eds.), Current concepts in clinical nursing. St. Louis: C. V. Mosby Company, 1967, 292-310.

200. Rutherford, J. Case conference 5: The young child in hospital. Nursing Times, 1963, 59, 1215-1256.

201. Saren, M. Viewpoints on children in hospitals: Administrator. Hospitals, 1963, 37, 49-52.

202. Sauer, J. E., Jr. Preadmission orientation: Effect on patient manageability. Hospital Topics, 1968, 46(3), 79-83.

203. Scahill, M. Preparing children for procedures and operations. Nursing Outlook, 1969, 17(6), 36-38.

204. Schaffer, A. J. Advantages of mother living in with her hospitalized child. In J. A. Haller, Jr. (Ed.), The hospitalized child and his family. Baltimore: Johns Hopkins Press, 1967, 33-41.

205. Schaffer, H. R. Activity level as a constitutional determinant of infantile reaction to deprivation. Child Development, 1966, 595-602.

206. Schneider, G. E. "Oliver" on the pediatric ward. American Journal of Nursing, 1968, 68, 2598-2600.

207. Schowalter, R. Parents are your patients too. RN, 1964, 27(5), 51-53.

208. Schowalter, J. E., & Lord, R. D. Admission to an adolescent ward. Pediatrics, 1969, 44(6), 1009-1011.

209. Schowalter, J. E., & Solnit, A. J. Child psychiatry consultation in a general hospital emergency room. Journal of the American Academy of Child Pyschiatry, 1966, 5(3), 534-539.

210. Schrun, D. Improving medical care of the adolescent. Medical Record and Annals, 1962, 55, 170-172.

211. Schulman, J. L., Foley, J. M., Vernon, D. T. A., & Allan, D. A study of the effect of the mother's presence during anesthesia induction. Pediatrics, 1967, 39(1), 111-114.

212. Schuster, H. H. Critique: Children's recall of a preschool age hospital experience after an interval of five years. In M. V. Batey (Ed.), Communicating nursing research. Boulder, Colorado: Western Interstate Commission for Higher Education, 1968, 73-84.

213. Seidel, H. M. Educational needs and programs for the hospitalized child. In J. A. Haller, Jr. (Ed.), The hospitalized child and his family. Baltimore: Johns Hopkins Press, 1967, 53-65.

214. Seidl, F. W. Pediatric nursing personnel and parent participation. Nursing Research, 1969, 18(1), 40-44.

215. Sexton, H. M. Emotional preparation for hospitalization. American Surgeon, 1960, 26(5), 422-424.

216. Shah, C. P., Papageorgis, D., Robinson, G. C., Kinnis, C., & Israels, S. A study of the need for alternative types of health care for children in hospital: Parental attitudes toward day care. Pediatrics, 1969, 44(3), 338-347.

217. Shore, M. F. Summary and implications. In M. F. Shore (Ed.), Red is the color of hurting. Washington, D. C.: United States Government Printing Office, 1965, 83-87.

218. Shore, M. F., Geiser, R. L., & Wolman, H. M. Constructive uses of a hospital experience. Children, 1965, 12(1), 3-8.

219. Sipowicz, R. R., & Vernon, D. T. A. The psychological responses of children to hospitalization. American Journal of Diseases of Children, 1965, 109(3), 228.

220. Skipper, J. K., Jr., & Leonard, R. C. Children, stress, and hospitalization: A field experiment. Journal of Health and Social Behavior, 1968, 9, 275-287.

221. Skipper, J. K., Jr., Leonard, R. C., & Rhymes, J. Child hospitalization and social interaction: An experimental study of mothers' feelings of stress, adaptation and satisfaction. Medical Care, 1968, 6(6), 496-506.

222. Slamar, C. F. Behavioral interaction between a three-year-old child with burn scars and his nurse. ANA regional clinical conferences, 1967, Philadelphia/Kansas City. New York: Appleton-Century-Crofts, 1968, 211-218.

223. Smith, M. Ego support for the child patient. American Journal of Nursing, 1963, 63(10), 90-95.

224. Smith, R. M. Preparing children for anesthesia and surgery. American Journal of Diseases of Children, 1961, 101, 650-653.

225. Smith, R. M. Children, hospitals and parents. Anesthesiology, 1964, 25(4), 461-465.

226. Solnit, A. J. Hospitalization: An aid of physical and psychological health in childhood. American Journal of Diseases of Children, 1960, 99, 155-163.

227. Sparks, L. Humpty Dumpty goes to hospital. Canadian Nurse, 1968, 64, 34-36.

228. Stainton, C. Preschoolers' orientation to hospital. Canadian Nurse, 1964, 70, 38-40.

229. Stein, A. Observations on socioprofessional factors mitigating against the psychological care of hospitalized children. Mental Hygiene, 1964, 48, 424-431.

230. Stoll, C. P. Responses of three girls to burn injuries and hospitalization. Nursing Clinics of North America, 1969, 4(1), 77-87.

231. Susser, M. Play and the sick child. Lancet, 1969, 1, 369.

232. Taylor, F. M. The hospital care of children. Hospital Progress, 1964, 45, 77-81.

233. Thornton, M. A play group on a children's ward. Nursing Times, 1967, 63, 574-575.

234. Thorpe, H. S. Psychological needs of hospitalized children and indexing of letters. Pediatrics, 1969, 44, 305.

235. Tisza, V. B., & Angoff, K. A play program for hospitalized children: The role of the playroom teacher. Pediatrics, 1961, 28, 841-845.

236. Tucker, M. N. The school-age child learns about the hospital. Hospital Management, 1963, 95, 99-102.

237. Vernon, D. T., & Schulman, J. L. Hospitalization as a source of psychological benefit to children. Pediatrics, 1964, 34, 694-696.

238. Vernon, D. T., Schulman, J. L., & Foley, J. M. Changes in children's behavior after hospitalization. American Journal of Diseases of Children, 1966, 111(6), 581-593.

239. Vernon, D. T., Foley, J. M., Sipowicz, R. R., & Schulman, J. L. The psychological responses of children to hospitalization and illness: A review of the literature. Springfield, Illinois: Charles C. Thomas, 1965.

240. Vernon, L. J., Jr., & Wheeler, W. E. The care-by-parent unit. Pediatrics, 1969, 43(4, part 1), 488.

241. Vigliano, A., Hart, L. W., & Singer, F. Psychiatric sequelae of old burns in children and their parents. American Journal of Orthopsychiatry, 1964, 34(4), 753-761.

242. Vredevoe, D. L., Kim, A. C., Dambacher, B. M., & Call, J. D. Aggressive post-operative play responses of hospitalized preschool children. Nursing Research Report, 1969, 4(2), 1, 4-5.

243. Webb, C. Tactics to reduce a child's fear of pain. American Journal of Nursing, 1966, 66, 2698-2701.

244. Weinberg, S., Schonberg, C. E., & Grier, D. Y. Seminars in nursing care of the adolescent. Nursing Outlook, 1968, 16(12), 18-23.

245. Weiss, S. The use of occupational therapy in a pediatric setting. Clinical Proceedings, 1967, 23, 118-123.

246. Wessel, M. A. & LaCamera, R. G. Care by parent: Further advantages (letter to the editor). Pediatrics, 1969, 44(2), 303-304.

247. White, F. P. Keeping kids happy though hospitalized. Medical Economics, 1969, 46(4), 98-103.

248. Whitted, B. A., & Scott, R. B. The significance of a play program in the care of children in a general hospital. Journal of the National Medical Association, 1962, 54(4), 488-491.

249. Williams, J. K. The dynamics of parent-adolescent interaction during hospitalization and implications for nursing care. In B. S. Bergersen, E. H. Anderson, M. Duffey, M. Lohr and M. H. Rose (Eds.), Current concepts in clinical nursing. St. Louis: C. V. Mosby Company, 1967, 328-338.

250. Wilson, R. D. Correlation of psychologic and physiologic observations from children undergoing repeated ketamine anesthesia. Anesthesia and Analgesia, 1969, 48, 995-1001.

251. Wines, D. Architectural aspects of services for children. In M. F. Shore (Ed.), Red is the color of hurting. Washington, D. C.: United States Government Printing Office, 1965, 73-80.

252. Wolf, R. E. The hospital and the child. In A. J. Solnit and S. A. Provence (Eds.), Modern perspectives in child development. New York: International Universities Press, Inc., 1963, 409-418.

253. Woodward, J. M. Parental visiting of children with burns. British Medical Journal, 1962, 2, 1656-1657.

254. Woodward, J., & Jackson, D. Emotional reactions in burned children and their mothers. British Journal of Plastic Surgery, 1961, 13, 316-324.

255. Wu, R. Explaining treatment to young children. American Journal of Nursing, 1965, 65(7), 71-73.

256. Wu, R. Child development: A basis for nursing care. In B. S. Bergersen, E. H. Anderson, M. Duffey, M. Lohr and M. H. Rose (Eds.), Current concepts in clinical nursing. St. Louis: C. V. Mosby Company, 1967, 269-283.

257. Zola, L. K. The effect of separation from parents on the dependency of asthmatic and non-asthmatic children (Doctoral dissertation, Boston University, 1967). Dissertation Abstracts International, 1967, 28(5-B), 2152.

AUTHOR INDEX

SUBJECT INDEX

MIX
Papier aus verantwortungsvollen Quellen
Paper from responsible sources
FSC® C105338

If you have any concerns about our products,
you can contact us on
ProductSafety@springernature.com

In case Publisher is established outside the EU,
the EU authorized representative is:
Springer Nature Customer Service Center GmbH
Europaplatz 3, 69115 Heidelberg, Germany

Printed by Libri Plureos GmbH
in Hamburg, Germany